THE

COCONUT

MIRACLE

COOKBOOK

[previously published as *Coconut Lover's Cookbook*]

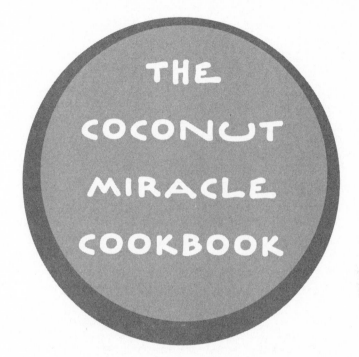

THE COCONUT MIRACLE COOKBOOK

Over 400 Recipes to
Boost Your Health with Nature's Elixir

BRUCE FIFE, C.N., N.D.

Avery
a member of Penguin Group (USA)
New York

Published by the Penguin Group
Penguin Group (USA) LLC
375 Hudson Street
New York, New York 10014

USA • Canada • UK • Ireland • Australia
New Zealand • India • South Africa • China

penguin.com
A Penguin Random House Company

Most Avery books are available at special quantity discounts for bulk purchase for sales promotions, premiums, fund-raising, and educational needs. Special books or book excerpts also can be created to fit specific needs. For details, write Special.Markets@us.penguingroup.com.

Library of Congress Cataloging-in-Publication Data

Fife, Bruce.
The coconut miracle cookbook : over 400 recipes to boost your health with nature's elixir / Bruce Fife, CN, ND.
p.   cm.
Previously published as *Coconut Lover's Cookbook* in 2004.
ISBN 978-1-58333-567-3 (paperback)
1. Cooking (Coconut)   I. Title.
TX814.2.C63F54   2014   2014022866
641.6'461—dc23

Printed in the United States of America
1   3   5   7   9   10   8   6   4   2

BOOK DESIGN BY TANYA MAIBORODA

Neither the publisher nor the author is engaged in rendering professional advice or services to the individual reader. The ideas, procedures, and suggestions contained in this book are not intended as a substitute for consulting with your physician. All matters regarding your health require medical supervision. Neither the author nor the publisher shall be liable or responsible for any loss or damage allegedly arising from any information or suggestion in this book.

The recipes contained in this book have been created for the ingredients and techniques indicated. The publisher is not responsible for your specific health or allergy needs that may require supervision. Nor is the publisher responsible for any adverse reactions you may have to the recipes contained in the book, whether you follow them as written or modify them to suit your personal dietary needs or tastes.

CONTENTS

1. Cooking with Coconut   1

2. Beverages   19

3. Salads   43

4. Sauces, Gravies, and Flavored Oils   59

5. Soups and Chowders   73

6. Main Dishes   95

7. Asian-Style Cuisine   115

8. Side Dishes   135

9. Breads and Grains   145

10. Cakes   165

11. Cookies   177

12. Pies   193

13. Puddings   215

14. Ice Cream   223

    INDEX   235

THE
COCONUT
MIRACLE
COOKBOOK

COOKING WITH COCONUT

Introduction

This book was written for people who love coconut. It was also written for the growing number of health-conscious individuals who recognize coconut as a marvelous health food and want to reap the many health benefits it provides.

Of particular interest is coconut oil, which has gained a reputation in recent years as a super health food. It is considered by nutritionists to be among the healthiest of all dietary oils. People who want to take advantage of the health benefits of coconut oil will find this book a blessing. It contains many creative ways to add the oil to the diet using a variety of delicious recipes.

Many people who live in non–coconut-growing regions of the world mistakenly think of coconut as just an ingredient for making desserts and sweets. Coconut, however, is very versatile and can be used in a variety of ways other than desserts. In this book there are recipes for creating savory main dishes, appetizing side dishes, satisfying snacks, and nutritious beverages. You will find a number of coconut oil– and coconut milk–based salad dressings that go well with both fruit and vegetable salads. You will also find recipes for creamy soups and hearty chowders, delicious curries, stews, and casseroles. You could literally eat coconut with every meal without consuming a single dessert. Of course, if you like desserts, you will find plenty here to choose from, including cakes, pies, puddings, and ice cream.

Every recipe in this book contains coconut in one form or another, whether it's coconut meat, milk, or oil. A large number of the recipes in this book, such as the Cheese Cups (page 142) and Sesame Chicken Salad (page 55), are completely original and found in no other source. Some of the recipes are variations on popular non-coconut dishes, such as Chicken à La King (page 108), using coconut milk in place of dairy. And, of course, this book wouldn't be complete without old favorites, such as Coconut Cream Pie (page 200) and Coconut Macaroons (page 177).

A Superior Health Food

Coconut oil is a uniquely curative elixir that has been shown to have countless health benefits. As a certified nutritionist and naturopathic physician, I've been recommending it to my clients for years. I've seen it get rid of chronic psoriasis, eliminate dandruff, remove precancerous skin lesions, speed recovery from the flu, stop bladder infections, overcome chronic fatigue, and relieve hemorrhoids, among other things.

Many people ask: Is coconut high in carbohydrate? If you're on a low-carbohydrate diet, you're in luck. Coconut contains very little effective (i.e., digestible) carbohydrate. Although coconut meat is mildly sweet, it is composed primarily of indigestible fiber and, therefore, is a low-carbohydrate, high-fiber food. Coconut milk, likewise, has very little carbohydrate, and coconut oil has none. For this reason, coconut is great for low-carb diets or for those who need to restrict carbohydrate intake.

Together, coconut meat and water contain a nearly balanced supply of nutrients, which are capable of sustaining a person with little additional food for extended periods of time. Coconut water, the juice in fresh coconut, has long been known for its healing powers and is recommended for those with digestive problems. For decades doctors in Asia have used fresh coconut water as IV solutions. Athletes now consume it because it helps replenish electrolytes lost in perspiration and to rehydrate the body. Among island populations, coconut water, coconut meat, and coconut milk have been used as both food and medicine for generations. Coconut in one form or another is used to relieve digestive problems, ward off infections, speed recovery from injuries, and maintain good health.

While the coconut is highly valued for its nutritional and curative properties, it is the oil in the coconut that makes it a truly superior health food. At one time, coconut oil had the misfortune of being labeled a dietary troublemaker because it is high in saturated fat. Many people avoided it for that reason. What most people didn't know at the time was that the saturated fat in coconut oil was a unique type of fat composed predominately of medium-chain triglycerides. This fat is completely different from the saturated fat found in meats and other vegetable oils and has a number of health benefits. Ironically, one of the benefits of coconut oil is that it helps *protect* against heart disease and stroke.

This fact is clearly evident in populations around the world who rely on coconut for food and eat it nearly every day of their lives. For thousands of years people in Southeast Asia, the Pacific Islands, India, and elsewhere have been consuming coconuts and coconut oil without any ill effect. In these countries heart disease is relatively rare. In fact, those people who eat the most coconut have the lowest heart disease rates in the world. Even though people in the coconut-growing regions of the world consume large amounts of coconut oil, heart disease was completely unknown to them until just a few decades ago. Heart disease didn't show up until after they began replacing traditional foods, such as coconut, with Western foods. Coconut was one of the key ingredients in their diets that protected them from heart disease as well as a number of other illnesses.

Coconut oil holds a high place of respect in traditional forms of medicine throughout the world. It is highly regarded in Ayurvedic medicine of India. In coastal Africa and South and Central America, coconut oil is a folk medicine used internally and externally to treat all types of health problems. In the Caribbean, coconut is considered a health tonic "good for the heart." In the coconut-growing regions of South America, people have a saying: "A coconut a day keeps the doctor away." Many Polynesian populations consider it the cure for *all* illness. Among the Islanders in the South Pacific, the coconut palm is so highly regarded, it is revered as the "Tree of Life."

In traditional forms of medicine, coconut oil is used to treat a wide variety of health problems ranging from burns and constipation to influenza and gonorrhea. Modern medicine is now confirming many of the benefits attributed to coconut oil.

Years ago it was discovered that human breast milk contained medium-chain triglycerides (MCTs). When eaten, the body transforms these triglycerides into powerful germ-fighting medium-chain fatty acids that kill disease-causing viruses, bacteria, and fungi. Researchers have determined that it is primarily the presence of medium-chain triglycerides in breast milk that protects infants from infections for the first few months of their lives. The medium-chain triglycerides in coconut oil are identical to those in human breast milk and contain the same germ-fighting properties. Research has shown that these coconut oil–derived fatty acids kill microorganisms that cause sinus infections, pneumonia, bladder infections, ringworm, candidiasis, influenza, measles, herpes, mononucleosis, hepatitis C, and many other illnesses. It's no wonder coconut oil has gained a reputation in traditional medicine as a miracle cure. Because of its germ-fighting potential, medium-chain triglycerides derived from coconut oil are routinely added to infant formula.

In addition to the germ-fighting properties, medical research has shown that medium-chain triglycerides also possess anti-inflammatory and antioxidant properties, all of which help protect the arteries from clogging up with plaque and the heart from succumbing to heart disease. This further confirms the observation that those people who eat lots of coconut oil have a low incidence of heart disease. For those who want to learn more about the healing miracles of coconut oil, I highly recommend my book *The Coconut Oil Miracle*.

Coconut oil can also help people lose excess body fat, increase energy, and improve thyroid function. Some people worry that if they add coconut oil to their diets, they will be consuming more fat and extra calories and end up gaining weight. In fact, just the opposite happens. The fatty acids in coconut oil are used by the body as a source of fuel to produce energy. Because coconut oil is used by the body as a source of fuel, it boosts energy and stimulates metabolism. This increase in metabolism, in turn, increases the rate at which calories are burned. So by adding coconut oil into your diet, you increase your energy level and burn off more calories. Simply adding coconut oil to a meal will lower the effective number of calories in the meal.

In addition, coconut oil has slightly fewer calories than any other fat. For these reasons, coconut oil has gained a reputation as being the world's only natural, low-calorie fat. Imagine that, a low-calorie fat that can help you lose weight! This is all backed by medical research. After I wrote *The Coconut Oil Miracle*, many people, most of whom had tried numerous other diets without success, gleefully reported to me their success at losing weight with coconut oil. Because of the miraculous results I saw, I wrote another book, *The Coconut Ketogenic Diet*. This book explains how to use coconut oil to raise metabolism, improve thyroid function, and lose excess weight. Both books are completely documented with numerous references to medical studies and success stories.

Recommended Amount of Coconut Oil

As I mentioned, most of the health benefits attributed to coconut come from the oil. For this reason, many people try to add as much of the oil into their diets as they can. I generally recommend 1 to 4 tablespoons (14 to 60 ml) a day, depending on your size. Three and a half tablespoons (52 ml) is a good maintenance dose for a 150-pound (68 kg) adult; however, you can still benefit from less. This calculation is based on the amount of medium-chain triglycerides a 7- to 10-pound (3- to 5-kg) baby receives from breast milk. The amount a baby receives is known to provide protection from illness, support good digestive function, and supply needed energy.

There is no danger of consuming too much coconut oil, except that if you're not accustomed to eating much oil, you may experience runny stools. I recommend that you add coconut oil slowly into the diet and combine it with your foods as shown in the recipes in this book. Start off limiting your coconut oil intake to 1 tablespoon (15 ml) per day. After a couple of weeks, increase it to 2 tablespoons (30 ml) a day, and continue in this fashion until you reach the level you feel comfortable with.

Many of those who use this book will want to prepare their foods so that they get a total of 3 to 4 tablespoons (45 to 60 ml) of oil in their meals during the day. As you prepare the recipes in this book, you can estimate the amount of oil you consume by how much you add to the food you eat. For example, if you add 4 tablespoons (60 ml) of coconut oil to a fruit smoothie, and the smoothie serves two, then you know that each serving contains 2 tablespoons (30 ml) of oil.

What if you use coconut meat or milk in place of coconut oil; how much oil would you be getting? You can determine that from the following table.

Approximate Amount of Coconut Oil Contained in Various Coconut Products	
PRODUCT OIL CONTENT	
1 cup (235 ml) coconut milk	3 tablespoons (45 ml)
1 ounce (28 g) fresh coconut meat	½ tablespoon (7.5 ml)
1 cup (78 g) dried, shredded coconut	3½ tablespoons (52 ml)

Coconut Products

The coconut is not really a nut; it's actually a seed. Unlike most other nuts and seeds, the coconut is the source of several food products. Besides the meat, you have coconut water, coconut milk, coconut cream, and coconut oil. In coconut-growing regions of the world, these products are used to make a variety of foods such as coconut wine, vinegar, butter, sugar, and more. Most of these more exotic coconut products are not readily available outside their native lands. The recipes in this book use coconut products that are readily available at your local supermarket or health food store. These products include coconut meat (fresh and dried), coconut milk and cream, and coconut oil. Coconut water is becoming increasingly popular, and a few recipes that use it have been included.

Coconut Meat

Fresh coconut makes a wonderful snack. You can eat it plain, or grate it for use in a recipe, or shred and dry it in order to store it in the fridge or freezer.

How to Choose a Good Coconut

Fresh coconuts are available at most grocery stores, health food stores, and Asian markets. The quality of fresh coconuts varies greatly even in the same store. The age of the coconuts and how they are handled greatly affects quality. Coconuts that have been battered around and cracked spoil very quickly. Once a crack occurs in the shell, mold quickly develops inside. Most coconuts are shipped long distances over extended periods of time. You have no way of telling how old they are when you buy them. The older they are, the more likely they are to be moldy.

You can identify mold when you break open the coconut and see yellow or brown coloring in the meat, or smell an off odor. Sometimes you can smell mold on the outside of the coconut before breaking it open.

When choosing a fresh coconut, look for one without any cracks. If the coconut is damp or has wet spots, it means the shell is cracked and the coconut water is leaking. Shake the coconut to detect the swishing sound of the coconut water. If there is little or no water in the coconut, it is old or cracked. Avoid those with white spots, particularly around the "eyes." The white is mold that has probably developed from water leaking from a tiny crack.

Even after you follow these guidelines, there is no guarantee that you won't get a moldy coconut. But at least your chances of getting a decent one are greatly increased. After you buy a coconut and bring it home, don't leave it on the countertop; store it in the refrigerator. The older it gets, the more likely it will go bad. So keep it refrigerated and eat it as soon as possible.

HOW TO OPEN A COCONUT

To open a coconut, first puncture *two* of the "eyes" and drain the water. Coconuts have three eyes. One of the eyes is soft and very easy to puncture; the other two are a bit more difficult. I use an ice pick. You may also use a hammer and nail. After draining the liquid, hold the coconut securely on a hard surface and hit it with a hammer. Coconut shells are very hard, so you will need to put some force into it.

Another way to crack a coconut shell is to place the coconut on a rimmed baking sheet and heat it in the oven for 20 minutes at 400°F (200°C). After it is heated, tap the coconut all over to loosen the meat, then crack it with a hammer.

Break the shell up into several pieces. With a table knife, you can pry the meat off the shell. The meat will have a brown membrane or skin on it where it was in contact with the shell. You can trim this off with a vegetable peeler, but it is safe to eat with this membrane attached. If you see any brown or yellow discoloration in the white meat, it is mold. Small patches of mold can be cut off and discarded. Most coconuts will have a spot or two. If a lot of discoloration is present, throw the whole thing away.

Dried Coconut

Dried coconut is sold under a number of descriptive terms such as desiccated, shredded, grated, flaked, and angel flaked. These terms can be confusing, especially since they are often used interchangeably. Therefore, it is important that you know what types of coconut to use in the recipes. In order to make recipes consistent and to avoid confusion, I use three terms to describe three different types of dried coconut. Because there is no standard terminology, these terms are not necessarily the same as those used by food producers or other cookbook authors. In this book, I refer to three types of dried coconut: flaked, shredded, and grated. When I say *flaked* coconut, I mean coconut that is in flakes. *Shredded* coconut is like what you would get if you used a grater to shred it. *Grated* coconut is very finely shredded or grated coconut. In essence, the difference among them is primarily size— flaked coconut being the largest and grated the smallest.

Most of the dried coconut in grocery stores is sweetened and contains preservatives. The recipes in this book use *unsweetened* coconut. If your local grocery store does not carry unsweetened coconut without preservatives, you can generally get it at your local health food store. Many of the recipes in this book call for grated or shredded coconut. If you don't have grated coconut available, generally shredded or flaked coconut will do. When measuring shredded coconut for recipes, do not pack the measure.

If you're using fresh coconut meat, you can make shredded coconut with a grater. One medium-size coconut will give you 3 to 4 cups (240 to 320 g) of fresh shredded coconut. Since most of my recipes call for dried coconut, you can dry your freshly grated coconut in a dehydrator or put it on a baking sheet in the oven for a couple of hours at low heat. Drying does not alter the nutritional value of the coconut meat; only water is removed. Dried coconut has a much longer shelf life than fresh coconut and will remain edible for a couple of months, or longer if you store it in the freezer.

Coconut Flour

Coconut flour is made from finely ground, defatted, and dehydrated coconut meat. It has a much higher fiber content than any other flour. It contains no gluten—the protein found in wheat and many other grains. Because of this, it is ideal for people who are sensitive to gluten or allergic to wheat. Although coconut flour doesn't have gluten, it does not lack protein. It has as much protein as whole-wheat flour. Coconut flour can be used to make a variety of baked goods including breads, muffins, cakes, pies, and cookies.

Coconut flour looks and feels much like wheat flour, but it doesn't cook the same. For this reason, you cannot use coconut flour in recipes designed for wheat flour. It just won't work. I do not include any coconut flour recipes in this book because coconut flour contains very little fat. The primary purpose of this book is to provide recipes that can supply a healthy dose of coconut oil to the diet. However, if you are interested in coconut flour recipes, I have an entire book devoted to this topic. It's titled *Cooking with Coconut Flour: A Delicious Low-Carb, Gluten-Free Alternative to Wheat*. If you are allergic to wheat, gluten-intolerant, on a low-carb diet, or just want to increase your fiber intake, you should take a look at this book.

DIETARY FIBER

Although fresh coconut is slightly sweet, it is a low-carbohydrate food. Coconut meat is composed mostly of non-digestible fiber with a fair amount of water and oil. It contains very little digestible carbohydrate. The fiber acts like a broom, sweeping the intestinal contents along the digestive tract, aiding in elimination and helping to reduce digestive problems such as constipation, colitis, and even colon cancer. Coconut meat is one of the highest natural sources of dietary fiber. I don't know of any food with a higher fiber content. It has more fiber than either oat bran or wheat bran and tastes a whole lot better! If you need to add fiber to your diet, coconut meat is an excellent way to do it.

Foods contain two types of carbohydrate: digestible and non-digestible. Digestible carbohydrate consists of starch and sugar and provides calories. Non-digestible carbohydrate is the fiber and provides no calories.

According to the U.S. Department of Agriculture, 24 percent of the carbohydrate in oat bran is composed of fiber. Wheat bran is 42 percent fiber. Soybeans contain only 29 percent fiber. Coconut beats them all. Its carbohydrate content is composed of a whopping 75 percent fiber!

Nutritionists recommend that we get 20 to 35 grams of fiber a day. This is higher than the average intake, which is about 14 grams a day. One cup of dried shredded coconut (unpacked) contains 12 grams of fiber. One 2 x 2-inch (50 x 50-mm) piece of fresh coconut contains 5 grams of fiber. Adding fresh or dried coconut to your diet can significantly improve your daily fiber intake.

Coconut Water

Contrary to popular belief, the liquid inside a fresh coconut is *not* coconut milk. This liquid is known as *coconut water* or *coconut juice*. Coconut water is a relatively clear, sweet-tasting liquid. Coconut milk, on the other hand, is manufactured by squeezing or extracting the liquid from coconut meat.

Coconut water is very different from coconut milk in taste, texture, and nutrient content. Because of its sweetness, coconut water is usually consumed as a beverage. It has a delicious flavor all its own and does not really taste like coconut meat. In addition to natural sugars, it also contains a complex array of minerals and electrolytes, which have made it popular as a natural sports rehydration beverage.

The electrolyte profile of coconut water is similar to human plasma, and for that reason it has been used by doctors as an intravenous solution and is injected directly into the bloodstream to prevent dehydration. Doctors working in tropical climates have often used the water from coconuts as IV solutions. This practice was common during World War II and in Vietnam, where commercial IV solutions were often in short supply.

The taste of coconut water varies depending on the age of the coconut. The water from fresh green (immature) coconuts is regarded as the best in taste and quality. The water from mature coconuts, although good, doesn't compare. Until recent years, just about the only way to get coconut water was to crack open a fresh coconut. Luckily for many of us, coconut water is now widely available commercially.

Because of its sweetness, coconut water can be used to sweeten other beverages such as fruit smoothies and blender drinks. Unlike most other coconut products, the water contains virtually no fat.

Coconut Milk

Coconut milk is made from squeezing the juice out of coconut meat. It is distinctly different from coconut water and has far more uses. This coconut meat extract has a milky white color, creamy texture, and nutty flavor. Coconut milk contains about 17 to 24 percent fat, which gives it its characteristic creamy taste and texture. Unlike coconut water, it is not sweet and, for this reason, can be used to make a variety of delicious soups, stews, sauces, curries, gravies, and desserts. Coconut milk can be used in place of dairy milk or cream in many recipes.

Canned coconut milk is available in many grocery and health food stores. It is most commonly sold in 14-ounce (400-ml) cans but is also available in larger cans as well as cartons. In addition to coconut milk, you can also find coconut cream, which has a slightly higher fat content. Don't confuse coconut milk or coconut cream with *cream of coconut*. Cream of coconut is coconut cream *with sugar added* and is very sweet. It is often used in beverages and desserts. Most of the recipes in this book use *unsweetened* coconut milk. If in doubt as to whether a brand of milk or cream has been sweetened, look at the ingredients label.

Some coconut milks have been watered down to reduce the fat content. This is called "low-fat" or "light" coconut milk. To retain the milk's thick texture, thickeners such as guar gum are added. I usually avoid low-fat coconut milks because the coconut oil content is reduced. One of the reasons I eat a lot of coconut is to get the benefit of the fat. I don't want to reduce the benefit by eating low-fat coconut milk. In my opinion, the higher the fat content, the better.

When canned coconut milk sits on a shelf for any length of time, the cream often separates and floats to the top, particularly with brands that do not add thickeners. To mix the cream, simply shake the can vigorously before opening. Sometimes you may want to separate the cream from the watery liquid. You would do this if you needed to use coconut cream in a recipe and had only coconut milk. In this case, don't shake the can. Open it and scrape the thick cream off the top. You can get more of the cream to separate by chilling the can in the refrigerator for a few days. The thickness of the cream varies from brand to brand, depending on the fat content and the presence of thickening agents.

Coconut milk spoils quickly after it has been opened. When stored in an airtight container in the refrigerator, it will last for about four days. If frozen, it will last for six months or longer.

Another type of coconut milk that has become popular in recent years is sold, not in cans, but in refrigerated cartons like dairy milk. Be aware that although the label reads "Coconut Milk," it is not real coconut milk like that sold in the cans; it is a coconut milk beverage. In other words, it is a manufactured beverage that includes coconut milk as one of its several ingredients. Water is the main ingredient and the beverage contains about 80 percent less fat. *Do not use this product in any of the recipes in this book!* It is meant for drinking and not for use in recipes that call for coconut milk.

Coconut Oil

You can use coconut oil in just about any recipe that calls for vegetable oil, shortening, butter, or margarine. Coconut oil is excellent for cooking. Unlike other vegetable oils, it is very stable when heated and does not create toxic by-products. You can feel safe when you eat it, knowing that you aren't damaging your health. Coconut oil, however, has a moderate smoking point when used for frying, so you need to keep the temperature under 360°F (180°C). If you don't have a temperature gauge on your stove, you can tell when it goes over this point because the oil will begin to smoke. This is a moderately high temperature, but you can cook anything at this heat, even stir-fry vegetables. When coconut oil is used to grease pans or in baked goods, it can be cooked in the oven at higher temperature because the evaporation of water in the food keeps the temperature at 212°F (100°C).

Because coconut oil is very stable, it does not need to be refrigerated. It will stay fresh for at least two and up to three years unrefrigerated. If kept in a cool place, its shelf life is extended. This makes it an excellent storage oil. I buy it by the gallon so that I always have an ample supply available.

Coconut oil melts at about 76°F (24°C), becoming a clear liquid that looks like almost any other vegetable oil. Below this temperature, it solidifies and takes on a creamy white appearance. At moderate room temperatures it has a soft, buttery texture and is sometimes called coconut butter. If your kitchen is cooler than 76°F (24°C), the oil will solidify. There is nothing wrong with this. Some people like to store the oil in the refrigerator. To liquefy the oil, simply immerse the bottom of the jar in hot water for a couple of minutes. The oil melts quickly.

Numerous processes are used to produce coconut oil, and the quality and taste of the oil vary from brand to brand. There are two basic types of coconut oil sold in stores: virgin and refined. Virgin coconut oil has had minimal processing and retains a mild coconut taste and aroma. Refined coconut oil is often labeled "expeller pressed" and has undergone more processing and is essentially flavorless and odorless.

Either oil can be used for any type of cooking or food preparation. Virgin coconut oil is preferred if you want to give foods a hint of coconut flavor. It generally is so mild that even moderately flavored foods will completely mask the coconut taste. For people who prefer not to have the coconut flavor in their food, expeller pressed oil is generally preferred. The way you can tell the difference between the two without opening the jar is by looking for the word "Virgin" on the label. All virgin coconut oils will proudly display this term in the title. Refined coconut oils can be labeled almost anything, such as "Expeller Pressed," "Natural," or "Organic," but will not include the word "Virgin."

A Note About the Recipes

As a nutritionist, I prefer to use the healthiest ingredients possible, choosing whole-wheat flour over white, brown rice over white, and natural sweeteners over highly processed or artificial sugars. I've made allowances in the recipes, however, for those readers who don't want to go all-natural.

Sugar and Sweeteners

You can use a variety of sweeteners for the recipes in this book, many of which are interchangeable. When the term "sugar" is used in a recipe, you can use white granulated sugar or any other *dry* sugar such as sucanat (dried sugarcane juice), date sugar, palm sugar, or dehydrated maple syrup. If the term "honey" is used in a recipe, you can substitute maple syrup, corn syrup, rice syrup, or any other *liquid* sweetener. A few recipes offer variations in which powdered stevia extract is used in place of either a dry or wet sweetener. This extract is a natural, noncaloric sweetener derived from the stevia herb.

Most of the recipes for sweets in this book include both full-sugar and reduced-sugar versions. So you can choose the one you prefer. Some of the reduced-sugar recipes use no added sugar, relying only on fruit, coconut, and/or stevia. Stevia is essentially calorie free. It is about two hundred times sweeter than table sugar, so only a little bit is needed to achieve the same level of sweetness. The major drawback with stevia is that if you use too much, it produces a bitter aftertaste. So for most recipes, you cannot replace *all* of the sugar with stevia. For best results, combine stevia with other sweeteners. This way, you can significantly reduce the total amount of sugar called for in many recipes. For example, you can reduce the sugar content in a recipe by half if you replace the other half with a little stevia. You will still achieve a sweet taste with only half the sugar.

If the recipe includes fruit, you can often eliminate all the sugar and use stevia instead. The fruit provides just enough natural sweetening to complement the stevia so that together they provide all the sweetness necessary.

A half teaspoon of stevia has the sweetening effect of 1 cup (200 g) of granulated sugar. If a recipe asks for 1 cup (200 g) of sugar, you can reduce the sugar to ½ cup (100 g) and add ¼ teaspoon of powdered stevia extract to achieve the same level of sweetness. When you substitute stevia for a small amount of sugar, be careful to use just a tiny bit. A little can go a long way and too much can give the food an overpowering aftertaste. If you are not accustomed to using stevia, it may take a little practice to find just the right amount to use to suit your taste. Stevia extract is available at most health food stores. No artificial sweeteners are used in any of the recipes in this book.

Concerned about sugar? No problem. All the dessert recipes can be made using natural sweeteners of your choice. In addition to the regular recipes, also included are reduced-sugar versions. Many of these recipes can be made with very little sugar or none at all. Some of the reduced-sugar recipes use stevia extract—a noncaloric herbal sweetener. Stevia makes an excellent noncaloric replacement for sugar or artificial sweeteners when used in combination with fruit and other naturally sweet foods.

Whole Grains

As a nutritionist, I strongly recommend the use of whole grains over processed, refined grains and flours. For this reason, the recipes in this book use whole grains whenever possible. When the word "flour" is used, I mean "whole-wheat" flour; however, if you prefer, you can use white flour in most of these recipes. When the word "rice" is used, I mean brown rice. In most cases you may use either brown or white rice. When it is important to use one or the other, a distinction will be made.

Serving Sizes

The serving sizes listed in the Nutrition Facts label on packaged foods and in most cookbooks are unrealistically small—½ cup in most cases. Who eats just ½ cup of spaghetti and meatballs or ½ cup (120 ml) of soup? An actual serving of soup is closer to 2 cups (475 ml). The serving sizes listed in this book reflect actual serving size—the quantity you would eat during a meal. The exception to this is when many small items are produced, such as pancakes or muffins. In these cases, a serving size is each individual item; 6 muffins would make 6 servings.

TERMS USED IN THIS BOOK

Unless otherwise noted, the term "flour" used in the recipes of this book refers to **whole-wheat flour**. All dried coconut used in these recipes is **unsweetened** and the coconut milk is **unsweetened.** The term "sugar" means any dry sweetener. "Honey" means any wet sweetener.

My Favorite Recipes

I like all of the recipes in this book. If I didn't, they wouldn't be here. While writing this book, I experimented with hundreds of recipes, adding and combining different ingredients to create a variety of appetizing coconut-based meals and beverages. Many of these recipes are completely of my own creation. Those that were based on existing recipes were usually modified to include coconut in one form or another. In compiling this book, I tried to include a variety of foods to suit a variety of tastes. A few, however, are my favorites. While we all have different tastes, I think most people would enjoy these just as much as I do. For this reason, I have included this symbol: 🌀 next to those recipes that are my favorites. I think you'll like them, too.

BEVERAGES

Homemade Coconut Milk and Cream

Commercially produced coconut milk and, to a lesser extent, coconut cream, are readily available at most grocery stores. This is by far the easiest way to get these products, but if you would like to try making the milk or cream at home from a fresh coconut, the following recipe will guide you through the process.

Fresh coconut milk, when refrigerated, and canned coconut milk, if not shaken, separate into two layers with the thick upper layer being the coconut cream and the thinner bottom layer the milk. The top layer can be skimmed off with a spoon and used for recipes requiring coconut cream and the bottom layer reserved for recipes specifying coconut milk.

You can get almost a quart (1 liter) of coconut milk from a single medium-size coconut. Drain the water out of the coconut and put the liquid aside. Remove the coconut meat. You do not need to peel the brown membrane from the flesh. Put the meat and 2 cups (475 ml) of hot water into the bowl of a blender and blend until the coconut is completely chopped. If you want the milk to be slightly sweet, use the coconut water you reserved from the coconut and reduce the amount of added water so that you have a total of 2 cups (475 ml) of liquid.

Over a bowl, press the contents of the blender through a triple thickness of cheesecloth or a fine-mesh sieve, forcing out as much liquid as possible. This liquid is the coconut cream and is very rich. The coconut pulp still contains a lot of juice that can be extracted. Put the pulp in a saucepan with 2 cups (475 ml) of water. Bring to a boil and simmer for 5 minutes. Let cool. Run it through the blender a second time. Press the juice out of the pulp using cheesecloth or a fine-mesh sieve. Discard the pulp or save it and use in other recipes to increase fiber content. Since the liquid from the second pressing will be less creamy than the first, you can mix the two together.

If you want a completely *raw* coconut milk, omit the step where you simmer the pulp in hot water. Run the pulp through the blender a second time and press the juice out as described.

If you do not use the cream or milk immediately, store it in an airtight container in the refrigerator. Use within two or three days. The cream and oil will separate out as it sits, so stir or shake well before using. The milk may need to be warmed to above 76°F (24°C) to completely dissolve the solids.

Another way you can make an unheated coconut milk or cream is to use a juicer. Juicing fresh coconut produces a rich coconut cream. This is by far the easiest way to make coconut cream. To turn the cream into milk, just dilute with a little water. Most juicers on the market, however, will not juice fresh coconut. Coconut meat is too hard on them. I know of only one juicer that can do the job and that is the Green Star juicer. The Green Star juicer has a powerful motor with heavy-duty twin gears that crush and pulverize the coconut. The cream is separated from the pulp with ease. The cream you get from this juicer is superior to any other and far better than the canned products you buy at the store. Since you make it yourself, you know it has no additives or fillers. Fresh coconut cream straight from the coconut is absolutely delicious!

Sweetened Coconut Milk

(An Excellent Replacement for Cow's Milk)

Fresh and canned coconut milks are naturally unsweetened, which makes them good for making soups and sauces where sweetness is not desired. Although many people enjoy drinking unsweetened coconut milk, most prefer a thinner, slightly sweeter beverage that more closely resembles cow's milk. This recipe produces an excellent nondairy replacement for cow's milk that can be enjoyed by the glass, poured over hot or cold cereal, or combined in a bowl with freshly cut fruit. This recipe makes about 2¾ cups (650 ml) of milk. Coconut milk spoils quickly, so keep it refrigerated and use within three or four days.

> 1 can (14 ounces/400 ml) coconut milk
> 1 cup (235 ml) water
> 2 tablespoons (40 g) honey, or more to taste
> Dash of salt

IN A MEDIUM BOWL, mix together the coconut milk, water, honey, and salt. For sweeter milk, add more honey. For creamier milk, use less water. Put in an airtight container and store in the refrigerator. Serve chilled.　SERVES 2

VARIATIONS

Adding 1 tablespoon (15 ml) of imitation coconut extract, vanilla extract, or almond extract can enhance the flavor of the Sweetened Coconut Milk. These flavors give the milk a wonderful added taste. It makes a great base for the Fresh Fruit–Flavored Milks (page 22).　SERVES 2

Coconut Water

Coconut water is the liquid that forms inside the coconut. Unlike coconut milk, which is made from expelling the liquid from coconut meat, coconut water is naturally sweet. The taste of coconut water varies somewhat according to the age of the coconut. The water from a fresh green (immature) coconut is very sweet and tasteful. The water from mature coconuts isn't nearly as flavorful. Because of its sweetness, coconut water can be used to sweeten other beverages such as fruit smoothies and blender drinks. Unfortunately, unless you live where coconuts are grown, it is difficult to get green coconuts. However, coconut water from green coconuts is now being commercially packaged and is widely available throughout the country.

Coconut Milk and Water Mix ✿

> ½ cup (120 ml) coconut milk
> ½ cup (120 ml) coconut water

COMBINING EQUAL portions of coconut water and coconut milk makes a deliciously coconut-flavored, slightly sweet beverage. It is excellent on hot or cold breakfast cereal, over fruit, or by the glass. It is a very healthy alternative to cow's milk. Use water from a fresh green coconut or a commercially packaged product for best results.   SERVES 1

Creamy Coconut Beverages

The following beverages use coconut milk as a base. Coconut cream may also be used if you desire a richer flavor and thicker consistency.

Fresh Fruit-Flavored Milks

The following recipes use the Sweetened Coconut Milk or Coconut Milk and Water Mix as a base in combination with fruits and flavorings to produce a variety of flavored milks. These milks taste great by the glass and can be used over hot or cold cereal.

Strawberry Milk ✿

> 1 cup (235 ml) Sweetened Coconut Milk (page 21)
> 1 cup (170 g) sliced fresh strawberries

IN THE BOWL OF A BLENDER, mix the Sweetened Coconut Milk and strawberries. Chill and serve. SERVES 1

Banana Milk

> 1 cup (235 ml) Sweetened Coconut Milk (page 21)
> 1 ripe banana, peeled and sliced

IN THE BOWL OF A BLENDER, mix the Sweetened Coconut Milk and banana. Chill and serve. SERVES 1

Mango Milk

> 1 cup (235 ml) Sweetened Coconut Milk (page 21)
> 1 fresh mango, peeled and chopped

IN THE BOWL OF A BLENDER, mix the Sweetened Coconut Milk and mango. Chill and serve. SERVES 1

Blueberry Milk

> 1 cup (235 ml) Sweetened Coconut Milk (page 21)
> 1 cup (145 g) ripe fresh blueberries

IN THE BOWL OF A BLENDER, mix the Sweetened Coconut Milk and blueberries. Chill and serve. SERVES 1

Apricot Milk

> 1 cup (235 ml) Sweetened Coconut Milk (page 21)
> 1 cup (165 g) chopped fresh apricots

IN THE BOWL OF A BLENDER, mix the Sweetened Coconut Milk and apricots. Chill and serve. SERVES 1

Kiwi Milk

> 1 cup (235 ml) Sweetened Coconut Milk (page 21)
> 2 kiwis, peeled

IN THE BOWL OF A BLENDER, mix the Sweetened Coconut Milk and kiwis. Chill and serve.   SERVES 1

Pineapple Milk

> 1 cup (235 ml) Sweetened Coconut Milk (page 21)
> 1 cup (165 g) chopped fresh pineapple

IN THE BOWL OF A BLENDER, mix the Sweetened Coconut Milk and pineapple. Chill and serve.   SERVES 1

Pineapple-Banana Milk

> 1 cup (235 ml) Sweetened Coconut Milk (page 21)
> ½ cup (82 g) chopped fresh pineapple
> ½ banana, sliced

IN THE BOWL OF A BLENDER, mix the Sweetened Coconut Milk, pineapple, and banana. Chill and serve.   SERVES 1

Piña Colada Fruit Drink

This drink can be made from freshly squeezed juices or from frozen concentrate.

> ¾ cup (175 ml) orange juice
> ¼ cup (60 ml) pineapple juice
> ¼ cup (60 ml) coconut milk

COMBINE THE ORANGE JUICE, pineapple juice, and coconut milk and mix thoroughly. Serve chilled.   SERVES 1

Creamy Fruit Punch

You can transform almost any fruit juice into a creamy delight with this simple recipe.

> ¼ cup (60 ml) coconut milk
> 1 cup (235 ml) fruit juice

MIX TOGETHER the coconut milk and fruit juice. Chill and serve. You can use almost any flavor of fruit juice available at your grocery store.   SERVES 1

Hot Chocolate

This is a great-tasting dairy-free chocolate drink.

> 2 tablespoons (12 g) cocoa powder
> ¼ cup (50 g) sugar
> Dash of salt
> 3 tablespoons (45 ml) water
> 1¾ cups (410 ml) coconut milk
> 1 teaspoon vanilla extract

IN A SMALL SAUCEPAN, mix the cocoa, sugar, and salt; stir in the water. Cook and stir over medium heat until the mixture boils; boil and stir for 2 minutes. Stir in the coconut milk and cook for about 5 minutes, until hot, but do not boil. Remove the pan from the heat and add the vanilla. Serve hot.   SERVES 2

Chocolate Almond ✿

> 2 tablespoons (12 g) cocoa powder
> ¼ cup (50 g) sugar
> Dash of salt
> 3 tablespoons (45 ml) water
> 1¾ cups (410 ml) coconut milk
> 1 teaspoon vanilla extract
> 1 teaspoon almond extract

IN A SMALL SAUCEPAN, mix the cocoa, sugar, and salt; stir in the water. Cook and stir over medium heat until the mixture boils; boil and stir for 2 minutes. Stir in the coconut milk and cook for about 5 minutes, until hot, but do not boil. Remove the pan from the heat and add the vanilla and almond extract. Serve hot or cold.   SERVES 2

Chocolate Mint

> 2 tablespoons (12 g) cocoa powder
> ¼ cup (50 g) sugar
> Dash of salt
> 3 tablespoons (45 ml) water
> 1¾ cups (410 ml) coconut milk
> 1 teaspoon vanilla extract
> ½ teaspoon peppermint extract

IN A SMALL SAUCEPAN, mix the cocoa, sugar, and salt; stir in the water. Cook and stir over medium heat until the mixture boils; boil and stir for 2 minutes. Stir in the coconut milk and cook for about 5 minutes, until hot, but do not boil. Remove the pan from the heat and add the vanilla and peppermint extracts. Serve hot or cold.   SERVES 2

Orange Cream ⚙

> ¾ cup (175 ml) orange juice
> ¼ cup (60 ml) coconut milk

MIX TOGETHER the orange juice and coconut milk. This produces a delightfully creamy orange drink. Serve chilled.   SERVES 1

Eggnog

> ¼ cup (60 ml) water
> 1½ tablespoons (20 g) sugar
> 1 teaspoon ground nutmeg
> 1 can (14 ounces/400 ml) coconut milk

1 large egg

Dash of salt

1 tablespoon (15 ml) vanilla extract

½ teaspoon almond extract

IN A SMALL SAUCEPAN, combine the water and sugar. Bring to a boil over medium heat. Stir in the nutmeg, remove the pan from the heat, and let the mixture cool for 1 minute. In the bowl of a standing mixer, combine the water mixture with the coconut milk. Add the egg, salt, vanilla, and almond extract and beat thoroughly on medium speed. Or combine the ingredients in the bowl of a blender and blend until thoroughly mixed. Chill and serve.
SERVES 2

Cinnamon Eggnog

¼ cup (60 ml) water

1½ tablespoons (20 g) sugar

1 teaspoon ground cinnamon

¼ teaspoon ground nutmeg

1 can (14 ounces/400 ml) coconut milk

1 large egg

Dash of salt

1 tablespoon (15 ml) vanilla extract

½ teaspoon almond extract

IN A SMALL SAUCEPAN, place the water and sugar. Bring to a boil over medium heat and boil for about 3 minutes. Stir the cinnamon and nutmeg into the hot water, remove the pan from the heat, and let the mixture cool for 1 minute. In the bowl of a standing mixture, combine the water mixture and the coconut milk. Add the egg, salt, vanilla, and almond extract and beat thoroughly at medium speed. Or combine the ingredients in the bowl of a blender and blend until thoroughly mixed. Chill and serve.   SERVES 2

Vanilla Cream

> ¼ cup (60 ml) water
> 1½ tablespoons (25 g) firmly packed dark brown sugar or
>   maple syrup
> 1 can (14 ounces/400 ml) coconut milk
> Dash of salt
> 1 tablespoon (15 ml) vanilla extract
> 1 large egg (optional)

IN THE BOWL of a standing mixer, combine the water, brown sugar, coconut milk, salt, vanilla, and egg, if using, and beat thoroughly on medium speed. Or combine the ingredients in the bowl of a blender and blend until thoroughly mixed. Chill and serve.   SERVES 2

Peppermint Cream

> ¼ cup (60 ml) water
> 1½ tablespoons (20 g) sugar
> 1 can (14 ounces/400 ml) coconut milk
> Dash of salt
> 1 tablespoon (15 ml) vanilla extract
> ½ teaspoon peppermint extract
> 1 large egg (optional)

IN THE BOWL of a standing mixer, combine the water, sugar, coconut milk, salt, vanilla, peppermint extract, and egg, if using, and beat thoroughly on medium speed. Or combine the ingredients in the bowl of a blender and blend until thoroughly mixed. Chill and serve.   SERVES 2

Vegetable Drinks

Coconut milk naturally goes well with fruit drinks. Vegetable drinks, however, aren't as compatible. The following drinks do not use coconut milk but do include coconut oil. These drinks serve as a convenient way to add health-promoting coconut oil to the diet without adding sugar or sweet fruits.

Tomato Juice Cocktail ⚙

This drink is good served hot and tastes much like a light tomato soup. It goes well with coconut oil, making it a convenient way of adding the oil into the diet.

> 1 can (8 ounces/235 ml) tomato sauce
> 1½ cups (355 ml) water
> ¼ teaspoon onion powder
> 1½ teaspoons freshly squeezed lemon juice
> 2 tablespoons (30 ml) coconut oil
> ¼ teaspoon salt
> Freshly ground black pepper to taste

IN A SMALL SAUCEPAN, combine the tomato sauce, water, and onion powder. Heat over medium heat until hot. Remove the pan from the heat. Stir in the lemon juice and coconut oil. Add the salt and pepper to taste. Stir and enjoy.   SERVES 2 TO 3

Snappy Tomato Juice Cocktail

This is a spiced-up version of the Tomato Juice Cocktail. It has a little more flavor and a bit of a kick.

> 1 can (8 ounces/235 ml) tomato sauce
> 1½ cups (355 ml) water
> ½ teaspoon onion powder
> Dash or two of cayenne pepper
> ¼ teaspoon garlic powder
> ¼ teaspoon paprika
> 1½ teaspoons freshly squeezed lemon juice
> 2 tablespoons (30 ml) coconut oil
> ¼ teaspoon salt
> Freshly ground black pepper to taste

IN A SMALL SAUCEPAN, combine the tomato sauce, water, onion powder, cayenne, garlic powder, and paprika. Bring to a boil over medium heat, then reduce the heat to medium-low and simmer for 1 minute. Remove the pan from the heat and stir in the lemon juice and coconut oil. Add the salt and pepper. Stir and enjoy.   SERVES 2 TO 3

Tex-Mex Tomato Juice Cocktail

This spicy drink has a bit of a kick to it.

> ½ cup (122 g) tomato sauce
> ½ cup (130 g) salsa
> 1½ cups (355 ml) water
> ¼ teaspoon chili powder
> 1 teaspoon freshly squeezed lemon juice
> 2 tablespoons (30 ml) coconut oil
> ¼ teaspoon salt
> Freshly ground black pepper to taste

IN A SMALL SAUCEPAN, combine the tomato sauce, salsa, water, and chili powder. Heat just to boiling over medium heat. Remove the pan from the heat and stir in the lemon juice and coconut oil. Add the salt and pepper. Stir and enjoy.   SERVES 2 TO 3

Shrimp Cocktail Drink ✿

> 1½ cups (355 ml) water
> ½ cup (113 g) cooked shrimp
> ½ teaspoon onion powder
> 1 can (8 ounces/245 g) tomato sauce
> 1 teaspoon freshly squeezed lemon juice
> 1 teaspoon chopped fresh cilantro
> 2 tablespoons (30 ml) coconut oil
> Salt and freshly ground black pepper to taste

IN A SMALL SAUCEPAN, combine the water, shrimp, and onion powder. Heat over medium heat until hot, about 5 minutes, then reduce the heat to medium-low and simmer for 1 minute. Remove the pan from the heat and add the tomato sauce, lemon juice, and cilantro. Transfer the mixture to the bowl of a blender and blend until thoroughly combined. Stir in the coconut oil, salt, and pepper. Serve warm.   SERVES 2 TO 3

Smoothies and Blender Drinks

There are as many smoothie recipes as there are people who make them. The combinations are nearly endless. There are no rules for making smoothies, and virtually any combination of fruits can produce a delicious-tasting beverage. Experimenting with different ingredients adds variety and adventure to the experience. Fruit smoothies are generally made with a liquid base such as milk or fruit juice with some combination of fresh or frozen fruits. Vegetables, vitamin and mineral supplements, wheat bran, seeds and nuts, and a variety of other ingredients are often added for their nutritional or health properties.

The liquid you use as a base for your smoothie can be milk, juice, or, my favorite, coconut milk or coconut cream. Another liquid you can use is coconut water. Being naturally sweet, coconut water will sweeten up any smoothie, eliminating the need for added sweeteners.

Because fruit is a primary ingredient, most smoothies are sweet. The level of sweetness depends on the ingredients you use and your taste. Some smoothies have added sweeteners while others rely only on the fruits or juice for sweetness. When sour (or unripe) fruits, unsweetened yogurt, or other ingredients are used, the smoothie often needs a little sweetening. You can use any sweetener of your choice, including stevia. If you don't like to use processed sweeteners, you can add apple or grape juice, well-ripened bananas, pineapple, raisins, or dates.

Raisins make a nice natural sweetener. But you can't just add them in the blender because they don't chop up finely enough. In order for the raisins to blend well, they need to be softened first. Heat 1 cup (235 ml) of water in a saucepan to boiling, remove the pan from the heat, and add ¼ to ½ cup (35 to 75 g) of raisins. Soak the raisins for 1 hour. Another method is to soak the raisins in cool water for several hours or overnight. Blend the softened raisins with about 1 cup (235 ml) of liquid before adding any of the other ingredients. Once the raisins are chopped, add the remaining ingredients.

Smoothies can be very liquidy or as thick as milk shakes. I recommend that you use cold ingredients (except for the coconut oil and egg mixture described in Super-Healthy Blender Drinks on page 36). For a thick smoothie, peel and cut the fruit beforehand and put it in the freezer. Blend frozen fruit with cold juice, yogurt, or coconut milk. Coconut milk tends to thicken somewhat when chilled and makes a great thick smoothie. If your smoothie is too runny, pop it into the freezer for an hour or two. If it freezes too much, put it back into the blender. It will come out perfect.

The following recipes are just a few of the many smoothies you can make. Experiment by using different types of fruits and different combinations. Yogurt can add a delightful, creamy tartness to smoothies. You can use plain or flavored yogurt, whichever suits your taste. I like the plain as well as the vanilla- and maple-flavored yogurts because they combine well with just about any type of fruit.

Basic Coconut Milk Smoothie ⚙

> 1 large ripe banana
> 1 cup (235 ml) coconut milk
> 1 cup (235 ml) freshly squeezed orange juice

IN THE BOWL OF A BLENDER, blend the banana, coconut milk, and orange juice until smooth. This smoothie recipe can be used as the base for many different flavors. (Coconut oil can be added if desired; follow the directions as described on page 37.) SERVES 2

FRUIT-COCONUT MILK SMOOTHIE
Make the Basic Coconut Milk Smoothie (above) and add 1 to 2 cups of any of the following fresh fruits: raspberries, blackberries, boysenberries, tart

cherries, pineapple, peaches, apricots, mango, papaya, strawberries, kiwi, or nectarines.

Tropical Fruit Smoothie

1 cup (165 g) sliced fresh mango
1 cup (165 g) chopped fresh pineapple
1 ripe banana
Freshly squeezed juice of 1 lime
1 cup (235 ml) coconut milk
4 ice cubes

CHILL ALL of the fruit and the coconut milk before starting. In the bowl of a blender, add the mango, pineapple, banana, lime juice, coconut milk, and ice cubes and blend until smooth. SERVES 3

Zesty Peach Smoothie

2 ripe peaches, pitted and peeled
¾ cup (175 ml) freshly squeeze orange juice
½ cup (120 ml) coconut milk
½ teaspoon ground cinnamon
⅛ teaspoon ground ginger

CHILL THE LIQUIDS and the peaches before starting. The peaches can be prepared beforehand and frozen if desired. In the bowl of a blender, add the peaches, orange juice, coconut milk, cinnamon, and ginger and blend until smooth. SERVES 2 TO 3

Yogurt Smoothie ✿

¼ to ½ cup (35 to 75 g) raisins, or use another sweetener
1 cup (235 ml) freshly squeezed orange juice
1 cup (235 ml) coconut milk
1 cup (230 g) plain yogurt
1 banana

SOAK THE RAISINS for at least 1 hour in hot water or in cool water overnight. When ready to make the smoothie, drain the raisins. In the bowl of a blender, add the raisins and 1 cup of the orange juice and blend until the raisins are pulverized. Add the coconut milk, yogurt, and banana and blend until smooth.   SERVES 3

Cherry-Yogurt Smoothie

1 cup (235 ml) coconut milk
½ cup (115 g) plain yogurt
1 ripe banana
2 cups (310 g) pitted fresh cherries
⅛ teaspoon almond extract
4 ice cubes
2 tablespoons (10 g) grated coconut (optional)

CHILL ALL OF THE INGREDIENTS before using. In the bowl of a blender, add the coconut milk, yogurt, banana, cherries, almond extract, and ice cubes and blend until smooth. For added fiber, you can add grated coconut.
SERVES 3 TO 4

Chocolate Fruit Smoothie

This is a thick, rich flavored drink that, when frozen, tastes a lot like ice cream.

2 ripe bananas
1 cup (255 g) fresh strawberries
¼ cup (60 ml) water
1½ tablespoons (20 g) sugar or sweetener of your choice
¼ cup (24 g) cocoa powder
Dash of salt
1 cup (235 ml) coconut milk
¼ teaspoon vanilla extract

PEEL AND SLICE THE BANANAS. Slice the strawberries. Freeze the bananas and strawberries overnight. In a medium saucepan, combine the water, sugar, cocoa, and salt and bring the mixture to a boil over medium heat, stirring constantly. Reduce the heat to low and simmer for 2 minutes. Stir in the coconut milk. Remove the pan from the heat, add the vanilla, cool the mixture, and place it in the refrigerator until chilled, at least 1 hour. In the bowl of a blender, combine the chocolate mixture, frozen bananas, and frozen strawberries and blend until smooth. For a thinner smoothie, add a little more water. SERVES 3

CHOCOLATE PEANUT BUTTER SMOOTHIE

MAKE THE CHOCOLATE Fruit Smoothie above as directed, but omit the strawberries and add ¼ cup (65 g) peanut butter. Almond butter can be used in place of peanut butter if desired.

Piña Colada Smoothie

This drink uses coconut water.

> 1 cup (235 ml) coconut milk
> 1 cup (235 ml) coconut water
> 1 cup (165 g) chopped fresh pineapple
> 1 banana

CHILL ALL OF THE INGREDIENTS, including the banana, before using. In the bowl of a blender, combine the coconut milk, coconut water, pineapple, and banana and blend until smooth. SERVES 3

Citrus Refresher

This drink is made with coconut water.

> 1 cup (235 ml) coconut milk
> 1 cup (235 ml) coconut water
> 1 banana

> 1½ cups (355 ml) freshly squeezed orange juice (juice from 2 fresh oranges)
>
> ¼ cup (60 ml) freshly squeezed lime juice (juice from 2 fresh limes)

CHILL ALL OF THE INGREDIENTS, including the banana, before using. In the bowl of a blender, combine the coconut milk, coconut water, banana, orange juice, and lime juice and blend until smooth.   SERVES 3 TO 4

Creamy Peach Smoothie

This drink uses coconut water.

> 1 cup (235 ml) coconut milk
>
> 1 cup (235 ml) coconut water
>
> 4 peaches, pitted and peeled
>
> ¼ teaspoon almond extract
>
> ¼ cup (36 g) almonds (optional)

CHILL THE COCONUT MILK, coconut water, and peaches before using. In the bowl of a blender, combine the coconut milk, coconut water, peaches, almond extract, and almonds, if using, and blend until smooth.   SERVES 3

Super-Healthy Blender Drinks

Smoothies and blender drinks made from fresh fruits and vegetables provide a good source of vitamins, minerals, and fiber. When coconut oil is added, the nutritional value greatly increases. Coconut oil provides many health benefits. It aids the body in fighting off infections, improves digestive function, and increases metabolism and energy level. In order to experience noticeable improvement in health and well-being, nutritionists usually recommend that adults get 2 to 4 tablespoons (30 to 60 ml) of coconut oil a day. Some doctors recommend up to 6 tablespoons (90 ml) a day for their sick patients.

One cup (235 ml) of coconut milk or coconut cream contains approximately 3 tablespoons (45 ml) of coconut oil. So if you use 1 cup (235 ml) of coconut milk in your smoothie, you will get the equivalent of 3 tablespoons (45 ml) of coconut oil.

If you want to increase the oil content of a smoothie without adding more coconut milk, you can. Simply mix together the coconut milk and coconut oil in the blender *before* adding any other ingredients. This works best if the coconut milk is at room temperature and the oil is melted. As much as 2 tablespoons (30 ml) of coconut oil can be easily blended into 1 cup (235 ml) of coconut milk. Combining the coconut milk and coconut oil will produce a cup (235 ml) of coconut milk with the equivalent of 4 tablespoons (60 ml) of oil.

When you add coconut oil to a smoothie, it *must* be mixed with coconut milk first. The other ingredients are added afterward. The problem with adding coconut oil later is that the oil solidifies at temperatures below 76°F (24°C). This explains why coconut oil sitting in a jar in your kitchen can be liquid one day and solid the next. If the temperature in your kitchen is above 76°F (24°C), the oil will be liquid. If you add melted coconut oil to a cold smoothie consisting of ingredients right out of the refrigerator or freezer, the oil will harden as soon as it hits the mixture. The blender will not blend the oil but will chop it into little chunks or beads, which many people find unappetizing.

Another problem with adding coconut oil to smoothies, and especially blender drinks and juices, is that oil and water don't mix. The oil separates and floats to the top. This problem is easily solved if you add an emulsifier. Coconut milk can emulsify the oil if mixed together separately, as described above. However, sometimes you may want to add coconut oil to a smoothie or drink that does not contain coconut milk. What do you use as an emulsifier? Egg yolk serves this purpose very well.

I prefer to use whole *raw* eggs. If you use organic eggs, there is virtually no risk of salmonella contamination. If you are squeamish about eating raw eggs, hard-boil the egg first, then remove the shell and egg white. Put the cooked *egg yolk* in the blender with the oil. You can blend at least 6 tablespoons (90 ml) of oil with 1 egg. I generally use 4 tablespoons (90 ml) in a smoothie that serves two. After the egg and oil are thoroughly mixed, add the rest of the ingredients and make the smoothie as you normally would. The oil will be completely blended into the smoothie and undetectable. The egg and oil blend best if the egg is warmed to about room temperature. After the oil has been emulsified in the egg, cold and frozen ingredients can be added without a problem.

You can use the same method to combine coconut oil with blender drinks and fruit and vegetable juices. This makes a very easy and tasty way to get your daily recommended dose of coconut oil. You can combine 1, 2, 3, or more tablespoons of oil into any type of juice or beverage by emulsifying it first with an egg.

Raw eggs supply the highest-quality protein available in our diet and are packed with vitamins and minerals. If desired, you can also add dietary supplements, fiber, herbs, and other products to boost the nutritional value of the smoothie. Coconut oil combined with fruit, vegetables, eggs, and a variety of supplements makes a super healthy blender drink.

Mango Smoothie

> 1 cup (235 ml) coconut milk
>
> 2 tablespoons (30 ml) coconut oil, melted
>
> 1 cup (235 ml) freshly squeezed orange juice
>
> 1 fresh mango, peeled and pitted

IN THE BOWL OF A BLENDER, combine the coconut milk and coconut oil and blend. Add the orange juice and mango and blend until smooth.

SERVES 2 TO 3

Pineapple Smoothie

1 cup (235 ml) coconut milk
2 tablespoons (30 ml) coconut oil, melted
1 cup (235 ml) freshly squeezed orange juice
1 cup (165 g) chopped fresh pineapple
1 banana

IN THE BOWL OF A BLENDER, mix together the coconut milk and coconut oil and blend. Add the orange juice, pineapple, and banana and blend until smooth. SERVES 3

Coconut Oil Juice Mix

This is a basic recipe that will work with any type of fruit or vegetable juice.

1 large egg
1 to 6 tablespoons (15 to 90 ml) coconut oil, melted but not hot
1 to 2 cups (235 to 475 ml) juice of your choice

WARM THE EGG to about room temperature. You can do this quickly by immersing the egg in a cup of hot water for a couple of minutes. In the bowl of a blender, combine the egg and coconut oil and blend for about 10 seconds (1 cooked egg yolk can be substituted for the raw egg, if you prefer). Add the juice and blend the mixture for a few seconds. It's ready to drink and enjoy. If desired, you can add vitamins and other supplements to turn this drink into a nutritional powerhouse. SERVES 1 TO 2

Peach-Yogurt Smoothie

¼ cup (35 g) raisins, or more to taste
1 large egg
¼ cup (60 ml) coconut oil, melted
1 cup (235 ml) freshly squeezed orange juice
3 to 4 peaches, peeled, pitted, and sliced
1 cup (230 g) yogurt (plain, vanilla, or maple)

SOAK THE RAISINS for at least 1 hour in hot water or in cool water overnight. For a sweeter smoothie, use more raisins. In the bowl of a blender, combine the egg and coconut oil and mix until well blended, about 10 seconds. Add the raisins and orange juice. Blend until the raisins are pulverized, about 1 minute. Add the peaches and yogurt and blend until smooth.   SERVES 3

Strawberry-Banana Smoothie

> 1 large egg
> ¼ cup (60 ml) coconut oil, melted
> 1 cup (230 g) yogurt (plain, vanilla, or maple)
> 2 cups (290 g) fresh strawberries
> 1 banana
> 1 cup (165 g) chopped fresh pineapple

IN THE BOWL OF A BLENDER, combine the egg and coconut oil and mix until well blended, about 10 seconds. Add the yogurt, strawberries, banana, and pineapple and blend until smooth.   SERVES 4

Powerhouse Mango Milk

This is a novel substitute for dairy milk. It is nearly white in appearance and somewhat resembles milk. It has a mildly sweet, coconut fruit flavor. You can use it in place of milk on cold or hot cereal, drink it by the glass, use it as a liquid base for smoothies, serve it in a bowl with fresh fruit, and much more.

> 1 large egg
> 1 to 6 tablespoons (15 to 90 ml) coconut oil, melted
> 3 cups (710 ml) fresh or frozen mango juice
> 1 cup (235 ml) cold water

IN THE BOWL OF A BLENDER, combine the egg and coconut oil and blend. You can use up to 6 tablespoons (90 ml) of coconut oil, but 2 to 4 tablespoons (30 to 60 ml) are usually enough. Add the mango juice and water and blend together. Any type of commercial mango juice or juice combination will work, such as mango peach or mango orange. If mango isn't available, you can also get good results with peach or apricot juice.   SERVES 4

V-8 Juice Blend

> ¼ cup (60 ml) coconut oil, melted
> 1 large egg
> 2 cups (475 ml) V-8 Juice

IN THE BOWL OF A BLENDER, combine the coconut oil and egg (or you can used a cooked egg yolk) and blend for 10 seconds. Add the V-8 Juice (or you can use a vegetable juice blend made with your own juicer).   SERVES 2 TO 3

SALADS

Salad Dressings

Coconut Mayonnaise

Coconut mayonnaise made with 100 percent coconut oil tends to harden when refrigerated and so can be used only when freshly made. This recipe can be made ahead of time and stored in the refrigerator; it remains soft and spreadable even after being refrigerated. The secret to this mayonnaise is the addition of a little olive oil. If you don't mind your mayonnaise tasting like olive oil, you can use extra-virgin olive oil. If you prefer a more traditional or mild-tasting mayonnaise, I suggest that you use extra-light olive oil. Also, if you like your mayonnaise to taste more like traditional mayonnaise instead of coconut mayonnaise, use expeller-pressed coconut oil instead of virgin coconut oil.

>2 large egg yolks
>2 tablespoons (30 ml) freshly squeezed lemon juice
>1½ teaspoons (7 ml) prepared mustard, preferably Dijon style
>⅛ teaspoon paprika
>⅛ teaspoon salt, plus more as needed
>½ cup (120 ml) olive oil
>¾ cup (180 ml) coconut oil, melted

IN THE BOWL of a blender or food processor, combine the egg yolks, lemon juice, mustard, paprika, salt, and ¼ cup of the olive oil. Blend for about 60 seconds. While the machine is running, pour in the remaining ¼ cup olive oil and the coconut oil *very* slowly in a fine, steady stream. The secret to making good mayonnaise is to add the oil *slowly*. The mayonnaise will thicken as the oil is added. Taste and adjust the seasoning as needed.

MAKES ABOUT 1⅓ CUPS (400 ML)

Thousand Island Dressing

> ½ cup (120 ml) Coconut Mayonnaise (page 43)
> 2 tablespoons (30 ml) chili sauce or ketchup
> ¼ cup (60 g) pickle relish
> ⅛ teaspoon paprika
> Salt and freshly ground black pepper to taste

IN A SMALL BOWL, mix together the mayonnaise, chili sauce, pickle relish, paprika, salt, and pepper. Store in an airtight container in the refrigerator. This dressing remains soft when chilled.   MAKES ABOUT 1 CUP (210 ML)

Buttermilk Dressing

> ¾ cup (175 ml) Coconut Mayonnaise (page 43)
> ½ cup (120 ml) buttermilk
> 1 teaspoon dried dill
> ½ teaspoon instant minced onion
> ¼ teaspoon garlic powder
> ½ teaspoon salt
> Dash of freshly ground black pepper

IN A SMALL BOWL, mix together the mayonnaise, buttermilk, dill, minced onion, garlic powder, salt, and pepper. Put the bowl in the refrigerator and let sit for at least 1 hour to allow the flavors to blend before using.

MAKES ABOUT 1¼ CUPS (295 ML)

Vinaigrette

> ¼ cup (60 ml) extra-virgin olive oil
> ¼ cup (60 ml) coconut oil, melted
> ¼ cup (60 ml) apple cider vinegar
> 3 tablespoons (45 ml) water
> ½ teaspoon onion powder
> ½ teaspoon dried dill
> ½ teaspoon salt
> ⅛ teaspoon freshly ground black pepper

IN A SCREW-TOP JAR, combine the olive oil, coconut oil, vinegar, water, onion powder, dill, salt, and pepper. Cover the jar and shake vigorously until the mixture is well blended. Let it sit at room temperature for 1 hour for the flavors to blend. Store in the refrigerator. MAKES 1 CUP (225 ML)

Italian Dressing ✿

> ¼ cup (60 ml) extra-virgin olive oil
> ¼ cup (60 ml) coconut oil, melted
> ¼ cup (60 ml) apple cider vinegar
> 3 tablespoons (45 ml) water
> ½ teaspoon garlic powder
> ½ teaspoon onion powder
> ½ teaspoon dried parsley flakes
> ½ teaspoon salt
> ½ teaspoon dried oregano

IN A SCREW-TOP JAR, combine the olive oil, coconut oil, vinegar, water, garlic powder, onion powder, parsley, salt, and oregano. Cover the jar and shake well. Let it sit at room temperature for 1 hour. Store in the refrigerator. MAKES 1 CUP (230 ML)

Creamy Coconut Dressing ⚙

This dressing is great for fruit salads or fruit and vegetable salad combinations. It has a mild sweetness that enhances the natural sweetness of fresh fruits and vegetables. Any of the four "C" Dressings (Coconut, Cinnamon, Cardamom, and Curry) can be used interchangeably in the recipes that follow.

> 1 cup (235 ml) coconut milk
> 1 tablespoon (8 g) cornstarch
> 1½ teaspoons (10 g) honey
> Dash of salt

IN A SMALL SAUCEPAN, mix together the coconut milk and cornstarch until blended. Add the honey and salt. Cook over low or medium-low heat, stirring constantly, for about 5 minutes, or until the mixture thickens and all of the taste of the cornstarch is gone. Remove the pan from the heat and allow the mixture to cool. Mix the dressing and chill. The dressing can be made ahead of time and stored in the refrigerator until ready to use.

MAKES 1 CUP (250 ML)

CREAMY CINNAMON DRESSING

Make the Creamy Coconut Dressing as directed above and add 1 teaspoon of cinnamon with the cornstarch. This makes a great-tasting dressing for fruit salads.

CREAMY CARDAMOM DRESSING

Make the Creamy Coconut Dressing as directed above and add 1 teaspoon of cardamom with the cornstarch. This dressing adds a unique flavor to salads.

CREAMY CURRY DRESSING

Make the Creamy Coconut Dressing as directed above and add 1 teaspoon of curry powder with the cornstarch. This mildly spicy dressing adds a pleasant kick to fruit and vegetable salads.

Mango Dressing

This dressing is a spicy blend of sweet and sour that goes well with both fruit and vegetable salads.

> 1 fresh mango, chopped
> ½ cup (120 ml) coconut milk
> 2 tablespoons (30 ml) rice vinegar or 1 tablespoon (15 ml) white wine vinegar
> 2 tablespoons (30 ml) freshly squeezed lime juice
> 1 teaspoon paprika
> 1 tablespoon (20 g) sucanat or honey
> ⅛ teaspoon salt
> Dash of cayenne pepper

IN THE BOWL OF A BLENDER, place the mango, coconut milk, vinegar, lime juice, paprika, sucanat, salt, and cayenne pepper and puree until smooth. Chill. The dressing will keep in refrigerator for about 1 week.

MAKES ABOUT 1½ CUPS (320 ML)

Sesame Seed Dressing ✿

This is an excellent dressing for tossed green salads.

> ½ cup (120 ml) coconut oil
> ¼ cup (36 g) sesame seeds
> ¼ cup (28 g) slivered almonds
> 1 tablespoon (15 ml) olive oil
> 2 tablespoons (30 ml) tamari sauce
> 1 tablespoon (15 ml) apple cider vinegar
> ¼ teaspoon ground ginger
> ¼ teaspoon salt

IN A SMALL SAUCEPAN, heat the coconut oil over low to medium-low heat. Add the sesame seeds and almonds and sauté for about 5 minutes, until lightly browned. Remove the pan from the heat and let the mixture cool to room temperature. Stir in the olive oil, tamari, vinegar, ginger, and salt. As the dressing sits, the oil will separate to the top and the sesame seeds and

almonds will sink to the bottom. Stir to recombine just before using. Spoon
the dressing onto the salad, making sure to include the sesame seeds and
almonds. MAKES ABOUT 1 CUP (220 ML)

Salads

Waldorf Salad ❁

> 2 medium apples, cored and diced
> 2 medium ribs celery, chopped
> ½ cup (60 g) coarsely chopped walnuts or pecans
> ½ cup (120 ml) Creamy Coconut Dressing (page 46)
> Mixed salad greens

IN A MEDIUM BOWL, combine the apples, celery, nuts, and dressing. Use
more dressing if you want a creamier salad. Stir well and serve on a bed of
lettuce leaves. Creamy Cinnamon Dressing (page 46), Creamy Cardamom
Dressing (page 46), or Creamy Curry Dressing (page 46) could be used with
this salad if desired. SERVES 2

Ambrosia ❁

> 1 cup (165 g) fresh pineapple chunks
> 1 can (11 ounces/260 g) mandarin orange segments, drained
> 1 medium apple, cored and chopped into bite-size pieces
> 2 medium bananas, sliced
> ¼ cup (35 g) raisins
> 1 cup (110 g) coarsely chopped pecans
> ½ cup (42 g) coconut flakes
> ¾ cup (175 ml) Creamy Coconut Dressing (page 46)
> Mixed salad greens

IN A LARGE BOWL, combine the pineapple, mandarin orange segments,
apple, bananas, raisins, pecans, coconut, and dressing. Use more dressing if you want a creamier salad. Stir well. Serve chilled on a bed of salad
leaves. SERVES 2 TO 3

Banana-Coconut Salad

This is a very simple, easy-to-make salad.

> **2 large bananas**
> **¼ cup (21 g) shredded coconut**

PREHEAT THE OVEN to 350°F (180°C). Peel and slice the bananas. Place the coconut on a rimmed baking sheet and toast in the oven for about 10 minutes, or until lightly browned. Mix together the coconut and banana slices. Serve fresh. SERVES 2

Tropical Island Salad

> **1 cup (165 g) chopped fresh pineapple**
> **1 banana, sliced**
> **1 orange, sectioned and cut up**
> **1 mango, peeled and sliced into bite-size pieces**
> **½ cup (42 g) shredded coconut**
> **¾ cup (175 ml) Creamy Coconut Dressing (page 46)**
> **Mixed salad greens**
> **Toasted flaked coconut**

IN A LARGE BOWL, combine the pineapple, banana, orange, mango, and shredded coconut. Add the dressing. Use more dressing for a creamier salad. Stir well and serve on a bed of mixed salad greens. Garnish with toasted flaked coconut. SERVES 2 TO 3

Raspberry-Banana Salad

> **1 envelope raspberry- or cherry-flavored gelatin**
> **2 cups (475 ml) Fruit Sauce (page 60) made with raspberries**
> **1 large banana, sliced**
> **Mixed salad greens**

MAKE THE GELATIN according to the package directions. Chill in the refrigerator for about 45 minutes, until partially set but still pourable. Fold in the

Fruit Sauce. Layer the banana slices on top of the gelatin mixture. Chill until firm, about 3 to 4 hours. Serve on a bed of salad greens.   SERVES 3

Creamy Melon Salad

> 2 cups (300 g) chopped watermelon
> 2 cups (320 g) chopped cantaloupe
> 1 orange, peeled and sectioned
> ½ cup (75 g) blueberries
> ¾ cup (175 ml) Creamy Coconut Dressing (page 46)
> Toasted flaked coconut (optional)

IN A LARGE BOWL, stir together the watermelon, cantaloupe, orange, blueberries, and dressing. Serve chilled with the dressing. If desired, top with toasted flaked coconut.   SERVES 2

Orange-Banana Salad

> 1 orange, peeled and segmented
> 1 banana, sliced
> ½ cup (120 ml) Creamy Coconut Dressing (page 46)
> Mixed salad greens
> ¼ cup (21 g) shredded or flaked coconut, toasted

IN A LARGE BOWL, mix together the orange, banana, and dressing. Place on a bed of mixed greens and top with toasted coconut.   SERVES 2

Cantaloupe-Cherry Salad

> ½ cantaloupe, cut into balls or cubes
> 1 cup (155 g) dark sweet cherries, pitted
> 1 cup (150 g) green grapes
> ½ cup (120 ml) Creamy Coconut Dressing (page 46), plus more to taste

IN A MEDIUM BOWL, mix together the cantaloupe, cherries, grapes, and dressing. Add more dressing for a creamier salad. Serve chilled.   SERVES 2

Summer Fruit Salad

1 cup (170 g) halved strawberries
½ cup (75 g) halved seedless grapes
2 medium peaches, peeled and cut into bite-size pieces
2 small bananas, sliced
¾ cup (175 ml) Creamy Coconut Dressing (page 46)
Mixed salad greens

IN A MEDIUM BOWL, mix together the strawberries, grapes, peaches, bananas, and dressing. Serve chilled on a bed of salad greens.   SERVES 2

Peach Salad

2 peaches, pitted and cut into bite-size pieces
1 cup (165 g) chopped pineapple
½ cup (120 ml) Creamy Cinnamon Dressing (page 46)
Mixed salad greens

IN A LARGE BOWL, combine the peaches, pineapple, and dressing. Serve chilled on a bed of mixed salad greens.   SERVES 2

Apple-Cinnamon Salad

2 apples, cored and chopped
¼ cup (35 g) raisins
½ cup (120 ml) Creamy Cinnamon Dressing (page 46)
Sliced almonds

PREHEAT THE OVEN to 325°F (170°C). In a 1-quart bowl, mix together the apples and raisins with the dressing and chill while you prepare the rest of the salad. Spread the almonds in a single layer on a rimmed baking sheet; bake for about 10 minutes, or until lightly browned. Allow the almonds to cool. Sprinkle the almonds on top of the salad just before serving.
SERVES 2

Carrot-Apple Curry

2 carrots, peeled and shredded

1 apple, cored and diced

¼ cup (35 g) raisins

¼ cup (about 33 g) walnuts or pecans

½ cup (120 ml) Creamy Curry Dressing (page 46)

IN A MEDIUM BOWL, combine the carrots, apple, raisins, nuts, and dressing. Serve chilled.   SERVES 2

Zesty Mango-Banana Salad

1 mango, chopped

1 banana, sliced

1 orange, sectioned

½ cup (120 ml) Creamy Curry Dressing (page 46) or Mango Dressing (page 47)

IN A MEDIUM BOWL, combine the mango, banana, orange, and dressing. SERVES 2

Tossed Curry Salad

2 cups (110 g) mixed salad greens

½ cucumber, peeled and sliced

½ green bell pepper, seeded and chopped

3 scallions (white and green parts), chopped

1 peach, pitted and cut into bite-size pieces

½ cup (120 ml) Creamy Curry Dressing (page 46) or Mango Dressing (page 47)

¼ cup (34 g) cashews, toasted

IN A MEDIUM BOWL, toss together the salad greens, cucumber, bell pepper, scallions, and peaches, and chill. Serve with the dressing, and topped with toasted cashews.   SERVES 2

Pineapple Curry

1 cup (165 g) chopped fresh pineapple

1 banana, sliced

¼ cup (35 g) roasted peanuts

½ cup (120 ml) Creamy Curry Dressing (page 46) or Mango Dressing (page 47)

IN A MEDIUM BOWL, toss together the pineapple, banana, and peanuts. Serve chilled with the dressing.   SERVES 2

Peach Curry

2 peaches, peeled, pitted, and cut up

1 banana, sliced

¼ cup (35 g) roasted peanuts or almonds

½ cup (120 ml) Creamy Curry Dressing (page 46) or Mango Dressing (page 47)

IN A 1-QUART BOWL, toss together the peaches, banana, and nuts. Serve chilled with the dressing.   SERVES 2

Peanut Butter–Apple Slaw

2 cups (140 g) shredded cabbage

1 cup (165 g) cubed fresh pineapple

1 apple, cored and chopped

¼ cup (21 g) shredded coconut

½ cup (130 g) peanut butter

½ cup (120 ml) Creamy Coconut Dressing (page 46)

Dash of salt

IN A LARGE BOWL, combine the cabbage, pineapple, apple, and shredded coconut. In a separate bowl, mix the peanut butter, dressing, and salt. Pour the peanut butter dressing on the slaw and combine all of the ingredients. Serve chilled.   SERVES 2 TO 3

Jicama-Mango Salad

1 cup (130 g) shredded jicama

4 scallions (white and green parts), chopped

4 cups (220 g) bite-size pieces of romaine lettuce or 1 10-ounce (68 g)
  bag mixed baby lettuce

¾ cup (103 g) roasted cashews

½ cup (42 g) shredded or flaked coconut

1 mango, pitted and chopped (see Note)

1 can (11 ounces/260 g) mandarin orange segments, drained

½ cup (120 ml) Mango Dressing (page 47), plus more to taste

IN A LARGE BOWL, mix together the jicama, scallions, lettuce, cashews, coconut, mango, and mandarin oranges. Keep chilled. Add the dressing just before serving. Add more dressing for a creamier and sweeter salad.

SERVES 2 TO 3

Note

You may use a peach in place of the mango if desired.

Potato Salad

6 medium red potatoes, cubed

1 cup (235 ml) Coconut Mayonnaise (page 43)

1 tablespoon (11 g) prepared mustard

¼ cup (60 ml) apple cider vinegar

½ medium green bell pepper, seeded and chopped

½ cup (50 g) sliced scallions (white and green parts)

2 ribs celery, diced

½ cup (72 g) chopped dill pickle

1½ teaspoons salt

⅛ teaspoon freshly ground black pepper

1 large hard-boiled egg, sliced, for garnish (optional)

IN A LARGE SAUCEPAN, place the potatoes and enough water to cover. Boil the potatoes over medium heat for about 20 minutes, until tender but still firm. Set aside to cool. Drain the potatoes. When cool, add the mayonnaise, mustard, vinegar, bell pepper, scallions, celery, pickle, salt, and pepper. If desired, a sliced hard-boiled egg can be added as a garnish. SERVES 6

HERBED POTATO SALAD

MAKE THE POTATO SALAD (page 54) as directed, but add ¼ teaspoon dried marjoram and 1 teaspoon dried dill.

Sesame Chicken Salad ⊕

This salad is so hearty and tasty, it should be eaten as a main dish.

> 1 cup (140 g) cooked chicken, cut into bite-size pieces
> 4 to 6 cups (220 to 330 g) mixed lettuce
> 4 scallions (white and green parts), sliced
> 1 tomato, chopped
> 1 bell pepper, seeded and chopped
> Sesame Seed Dressing (page 47)
> 6 to 12 Fried Wonton Skins (page 96) (see Note), for garnish

IN A LARGE BOWL, mix together the chicken, lettuce, scallions, tomato, and bell pepper. Serve in individual bowls and add dressing as desired. Break Fried Wonton Skins into bite-size pieces and sprinkle on top of the salad as a garnish. SERVES 3 TO 4

Note

You may substitute 1 cup (85 g) of toasted flaked coconut for the wontons if you desire. To toast the coconut, place on a rimmed baking sheet in a 350°F (180°C) oven for 8 to 10 minutes, or until golden brown.

Japanese Vegetable Salad with Sesame Seed Dressing

> 2 cups (110 g) mixed salad greens
> 1 cup (70 g) shredded or finely cut red cabbage
> 1 cup (135 g) peeled and shredded cucumber
> ½ cup (58 g) shredded radish
> ½ cup (55 g) shredded carrot

½ cup (133 g) minced cooked shrimp

¼ cup (60 ml) Sesame Seed Dressing (page 47)

IN A LARGE BOWL, place the salad greens, cabbage, cucumber, radish, carrot, and shrimp. Pour the dressing into the bowl and toss well to mix.
SERVES 2

Turkey Calypso Salad

½ cup (95 g) brown rice

¼ cup (41 g) wild rice

1½ cups (355 ml) salted water

1 cup (85 g) flaked coconut

½ red bell pepper, seeded and chopped

1 tablespoon (9 g) finely diced chili pepper

5 scallions (white and green parts), chopped

1 rib celery, chopped

1 tablespoon (1 g) cilantro

2 mangos or peaches, pitted and chopped

¼ to ½ pound (113 to 226 g) cooked turkey or chicken, cut into
　　matchstick strips

½ to 1 cup (120 to 240 ml) Orange Dressing (recipe follows)

IN A MEDIUM SAUCEPAN, combine the brown rice, wild rice, and water. Bring the mixture to a boil over high heat. Reduce the heat to medium-low and cook, covered, for 50 to 60 minutes, or until the rice is tender. Drain, if necessary, and cool. Preheat the oven to 375°F (190°C). Spread the coconut evenly on a rimmed baking sheet. Bake for about 10 minutes, until lightly browned, then let cool. In a large bowl, combine the cooked rice with the flaked coconut, bell pepper, chili pepper, scallions, celery, cilantro, mangos, and chicken. Mix with the dressing.　SERVES 2 TO 3

Orange Dressing

¾ cup (175 ml) freshly squeezed orange juice

2 tablespoons (30 ml) olive oil

1 tablespoon (15 ml) balsamic vinegar

½ teaspoon salt

⅛ teaspoon freshly ground black pepper

IN A SMALL BOWL, whisk together the orange juice, olive oil, vinegar, salt, and pepper. Store any leftover dressing in the refrigerator.

MAKES ABOUT 1 CUP (240 ML)

Coconut Rice Salad

½ cup (95 g) brown rice

1 cup (235 ml) freshly squeezed orange juice

2 tablespoons (30 g) sucanat or firmly packed dark brown sugar

⅛ teaspoon salt

1 teaspoon ground cinnamon

1 cup (235 ml) coconut milk

1 can (11 ounces/260 g) mandarin orange segments, drained

1 cup (85 g) shredded or flaked coconut, toasted

IN A MEDIUM SAUCEPAN, soak the rice in 2 cups water for 4 hours or over-night. Drain and add the orange juice, sucanat, and salt. Cook the rice and orange juice mixture, covered, over medium-low heat for 60 minutes, or until the juice is absorbed and the rice is tender. Remove the pan from the heat, stir in the cinnamon, cool, and chill the mixture for at least 2 hours. Mix the coconut milk and mandarin oranges into the rice. The salad will be somewhat runny and will need to be served in bowls. Just before serving, top generously with toasted coconut. SERVES 2 TO 3

SAUCES, GRAVIES, AND FLAVORED OILS

Sauces

Tartar Sauce

1 cup (235 ml) Coconut Mayonnaise (page 43)

3 scallions (white and green parts), minced

1 tablespoon (4 g) minced fresh parsley

1 tablespoon (4 g) minced fresh tarragon

¼ cup (60 g) dill pickle relish

2 tablespoons (17 g) capers

1 teaspoon prepared Dijon-style mustard

½ teaspoon sugar

2 tablespoons (30 ml) red wine vinegar

IN A SMALL BOWL, mix together the mayonnaise, scallions, parsley, tarragon, pickle relish, capers, mustard, sugar, and vinegar. Cover and chill. Serve with seafood. MAKES ABOUT 1¼ CUPS (295 ML)

Quick Tartar Sauce

> 1 cup (235 ml) Coconut Mayonnaise (page 43)
> ¼ cup (60 g) dill pickle relish
> 3 scallions (white and green parts), minced

IN A SMALL BOWL, mix together the mayonnaise, pickle relish, and scallions. Cover and chill.   MAKES ABOUT 1¼ CUPS (295 ML)

Guacamole

> 1 avocado
> 2 scallions (white and green parts), diced
> ½ teaspoon freshly squeezed lemon juice
> ⅛ teaspoon salt
> ¼ teaspoon onion powder
> ⅛ teaspoon chili powder
> 2 tablespoons (30 ml) Coconut Mayonnaise (page 43)

IN A SMALL BOWL, pit and mash the avocado with a fork. Stir in the scallions, lemon juice, salt, onion powder, and chili powder. Blend in the mayonnaise. Serve as a dip or spread.   MAKES ABOUT ½ CUP

Fruit Sauce ⚙

This is a great sauce to use as a flavoring for hot cereal; a spread on toast; a filling for crepes; or a topping on pancakes, waffles, and French toast.

> 1 tablespoon (8 g) cornstarch
> 1 cup (235 ml) coconut milk
> ⅓ cup (155 g) honey, plus more to taste
> Dash of salt
> 1 cup fruit (see note)
> 1 teaspoon freshly squeezed lemon juice
> ¼ teaspoon vanilla extract
> ⅛ teaspoon almond extract

IN A SMALL SAUCEPAN, stir the cornstarch into the coconut milk and mix until dissolved. Add the honey and salt. Bring to a boil over medium heat, then reduce the heat to medium-low and simmer, stirring constantly, for about 5 minutes, until thickened. Add the fruit and continue to simmer for 5 minutes. Remove the pan from the heat and add the lemon juice, vanilla, and almond extract. Taste for sweetness and add more honey if desired.
MAKES ABOUT 2 CUPS (500 ML)

Note

Use fresh or canned cherries, peaches, apricots, apples, strawberries, raspberries, boysenberries, or blueberries. If using peaches or apples, add ½ teaspoon cinnamon and a dash of nutmeg.

REDUCED-SUGAR FRUIT SAUCE

Make the Fruit Sauce as directed above, but omit the honey and add ⅛ teaspoon of powdered stevia or more for desired sweetness.

Coconut Sauce ⚙

This is a rich-tasting coconut-flavored sauce that goes well over pancakes, fresh fruit, rice, or desserts.

> 1 can (14 ounces/400 ml) coconut milk
> ½ cup (100 g) sugar
> ¼ cup (32 g) cornstarch
> ½ teaspoon imitation coconut extract (optional)

IN A MEDIUM SAUCEPAN, mix together the coconut milk, sugar, and cornstarch. Bring the mixture to a boil over medium heat, then reduce the heat and simmer for about 5 minutes, stirring constantly, until the mixture thickens. Add the coconut extract, if using. Remove the pan from heat and cool. Serve the sauce lukewarm. It can be stored in an airtight container in the refrigerator for about a week. MAKES ABOUT 2 CUPS (460 ML)

REDUCED-SUGAR COCONUT SAUCE

Make the Coconut Sauce according to the directions above, but reduce the amount of sugar to ¼ cup (50 g) and add a dash or two of powdered stevia.

Coconut Custard Sauce ✿

> 1 can (14 ounces/400 ml) coconut milk
> ½ cup (42 g) grated coconut
> 5 tablespoons (65 g) sugar
> Dash of salt
> 4 large egg yolks, slightly beaten
> ½ teaspoon vanilla extract
> ¼ teaspoon almond extract

IN A SMALL SAUCEPAN, place the coconut milk, coconut, sugar, and salt. Bring to a boil over medium heat, reduce the heat to low, and simmer for 5 minutes, stirring constantly. Remove the pan from the heat and slowly stir about half of the hot mixture into the egg yolks. Combine the egg yolk mixture with the rest of the hot mixture and stir. Return the pan to the stove and heat the mixture over medium heat for 2 to 3 minutes, until thickened. Remove the pan from the heat and add the vanilla and almond extract. This may be served hot or cold. It can be eaten as is or served over cake, pancakes, or fresh fruit.   MAKES ABOUT 2 CUPS (480 ML)

REDUCED-SUGAR COCONUT CUSTARD SAUCE

Prepare the Coconut Custard Sauce as directed above, but reduce the sugar to 2 to 3 tablespoons (26 to 39 g) and add up to ⅛ teaspoon of powdered stevia.

Cheese Sauces ✿

Cheese sauces make great toppings or dips for a variety of raw vegetables as well as French fries, corn chips, and crackers. They also make great toppings for cooked vegetables, pasta, baked potatoes, eggs, casseroles, and other dishes.

Creamy Cheese Sauce

This is the basic cheese sauce recipe. Variations are described below.

> 3 tablespoons (42 g) salted butter
> 2 teaspoons cornstarch
> ¼ teaspoon salt
> 1 cup (235 ml) coconut milk
> 1 cup (6 ounces/115 g) shredded sharp cheddar cheese

IN A SMALL SAUCEPAN, melt the butter over low heat. In a small bowl, combine the cornstarch, salt, and coconut milk and add the mixture to the saucepan. Stir constantly for about 5 minutes, until the mixture thickens and bubbles. Remove the pan from the heat and add the cheese, stirring for about 6 minutes, until melted. For a thinner sauce, add a little more coconut milk. MAKES ABOUT 1½ CUPS (360 ML)

THICK CHEDDAR CHEESE SAUCE
Follow the directions for the Creamy Cheese Sauce as directed above, but increase the cornstarch to 4 teaspoons and the cheddar cheese to 1¼ cups (145 g). This sauce is very thick and makes a good replacement for soft cheese in recipes.

TEX-MEX CHEDDAR CHEESE SAUCE
Make the Thick Cheddar Cheese Sauce as directed above, and add ½ cup (130 g) salsa.

GARLIC CHEESE SAUCE
Make the Creamy Cheese Sauce as directed above, but sauté 6 cloves of diced garlic with the butter. Use more garlic if you prefer a stronger flavor.

CRAB CHEESE SAUCE
Make the Creamy Cheese Sauce as directed above, but delete the salt and add 2 cans (7½ ounces/212 g each) of crabmeat as the mixture begins to boil. Cook for 1 minute longer, remove the pan from the heat, and add the cheese and 1 teaspoon of fish sauce (see Note).

Note
Fish sauce is available in the Asian section of the grocery store.

SHRIMP CHEESE SAUCE

Make the Creamy Cheese Sauce (page 63) as directed, but delete the salt and add 1½ cups (340 g) of baby shrimp as the mixture begins to boil. Cook for 1 minute longer, remove the pan from the heat, and add the cheese and 1 teaspoon of fish sauce (see Note).

Note

Fish sauce is available in the Asian section of the grocery store.

MUSHROOM AND ONION CHEESE SAUCE

In a medium saucepan, sauté 1 cup (70 g) of chopped mushrooms and ½ cup (50 g) of diced onion in 3 tablespoons (42 g) salted butter, olive oil, or coconut oil over medium heat for about 6 to 7 minutes, until tender. Make the Creamy Cheese Sauce (page 63) as directed, and add to the mushrooms and onions.

Gravies

Mashed potatoes and gravy are a traditional favorite combination. Gravy, however, isn't just for mashed potatoes. The gravies described below taste great combined with a variety of foods. Try them on pasta, biscuits, toast, steamed vegetables, and rice.

Vegetarian Gravy

½ cup (120 ml) coconut oil
⅓ cup (33 g) chopped onion
5 cloves garlic, minced
½ cup (62 g) flour
2 cups (475 ml) vegetable broth
3 tablespoons (45 ml) soy sauce
½ teaspoon dried sage
½ teaspoon salt
¼ teaspoon freshly ground black pepper

IN A MEDIUM SAUCEPAN, heat the coconut oil over medium heat. Add the onion and garlic and sauté for about 5 minutes, until soft. Stir in the flour and cook for 4 minutes. Add the broth, soy sauce, sage, salt, and pepper. Bring to a boil, reduce the heat to medium-low, and simmer, stirring constantly, for about 4 to 5 minutes, until thickened.   MAKES ABOUT 3½ CUPS (660 ML)

White Cream Gravy

3 tablespoons (42 g) salted butter
⅓ cup (33 g) chopped onion
5 cloves garlic, minced
3 tablespoons (23 g) flour
1 can (14 ounces/400 ml) coconut milk
½ teaspoon salt
¼ teaspoon freshly ground black pepper

IN A SMALL SAUCEPAN, melt the butter over medium heat. Add the onion and garlic and sauté for about 5 minutes, until soft. Stir in the flour and cook for 4 minutes. Add the coconut milk, salt, and pepper. Bring to a boil, reduce the heat to medium-low, and simmer, stirring constantly, for about 5 minutes, until thickened.   MAKES ABOUT 2 CUPS (450 ML)

Chicken Gravy ⚙

3 tablespoons (42 g) salted butter
⅓ cup (33 g) chopped onion
5 cloves garlic, minced
1½ tablespoons (12 g) cornstarch
1 cup (235 ml) coconut milk
1 cup (235 ml) chicken broth
1 teaspoon dried sage
½ teaspoon salt
¼ teaspoon freshly ground black pepper

IN A MEDIUM SAUCEPAN, melt the butter over medium heat. Add the onion and garlic and sauté for about 8 minutes, until soft and lightly browned. In a small bowl, stir the cornstarch into the coconut milk and mix until thoroughly dissolved. Add the coconut milk, broth, sage, salt, and pepper to the hot mixture. Bring to a boil, reduce the heat to medium-low, and simmer, stirring constantly, for about 5 minutes, until thickened.

MAKES ABOUT 2¼ CUPS (520 ML)

Curry Gravy

> 3 tablespoons (42 g) unsalted butter
>
> ⅓ cup (33 g) chopped onion
>
> 5 cloves garlic, minced
>
> 1½ tablespoons (12 g) cornstarch
>
> 1 cup (235 ml) coconut milk
>
> 1 cup (235 ml) chicken broth
>
> 1 teaspoon curry powder or garam masala
>
> ½ teaspoon salt
>
> ¼ teaspoon freshly ground black pepper

IN A MEDIUM SAUCEPAN, melt the butter over medium heat. Add the onion and garlic and sauté for about 8 minutes, until soft and lightly browned. In a small bowl, mix the cornstarch into the coconut milk until thoroughly dissolved. Add the coconut milk, broth, curry powder, salt, and pepper to the hot mixture. Bring to a boil, reduce the heat to medium-low, and simmer, stirring constantly, for about 5 minutes, until thickened.

MAKES ABOUT 2¼ CUPS (520 ML)

Sausage Gravy

> 1 pound (455 g) sausage
>
> ⅓ cup (33 g) chopped onion
>
> 5 cloves garlic, minced
>
> 2 tablespoons (16 g) cornstarch
>
> ½ cup (120 ml) water
>
> 1 can (14 ounces/400 ml) coconut milk
>
> 1 teaspoon dried sage
>
> ½ teaspoon paprika
>
> ½ teaspoon salt
>
> ¼ teaspoon freshly ground black pepper

IN A MEDIUM SKILLET, add the sausage, onion, and garlic and cook over medium-high heat for about 5 minutes, until the meat is browned and the vegetables are tender. In a small bowl, stir the cornstarch into the water and mix until thoroughly dissolved. Mix the water, coconut milk, sage, paprika, salt, and pepper into the hot mixture. Bring to a boil, reduce the heat to medium-low, and simmer, stirring constantly, for about 5 minutes, until thickened. MAKES ABOUT 4½ CUPS (1,000 ML)

SPICY SAUSAGE GRAVY

Make the Sausage Gravy as directed above, but omit the sage and add ¼ cup (65 g) of salsa. Add a dash or two of cayenne pepper if desired.

Chunky Chicken Gravy ✿

3 tablespoons (42 g) salted butter

½ cup (50 g) chopped onion

5 cloves garlic, minced

2 tablespoons (16 g) cornstarch

1 cup (235 ml) chicken broth or water

1 cup (140 g) bite-size pieces of cooked chicken

1 can (4 ounces/35 g) mushrooms

1 can (14 ounces/400 ml) coconut milk

1 teaspoon dried sage

½ teaspoon salt

¼ teaspoon freshly ground black pepper

IN A LARGE SAUCEPAN, melt the butter over medium heat. Add the onion and garlic and sauté for about 8 minutes, until soft and lightly browned. In a small bowl, stir the cornstarch into the broth and mix until thoroughly dissolved. Add the broth, chicken, mushrooms, coconut milk, sage, salt, and pepper to the hot mixture. Bring to a boil, reduce the heat to medium-low, and simmer, stirring constantly, for about 6 minutes, until thickened. MAKES ABOUT 4½ CUPS (1,000 ML)

Flavored Oils

Coconut oil generally has a mild flavor. Some brands are completely flavorless. The mild flavor makes the oil ideal for general cooking purposes, but it is often too bland as a spread or topping. A variety of flavors can be added to the oil to enhance its taste and aroma. Flavored oils can be used as a spread in place of butter; a dip for bread and chips; or a topping on meats, steamed or raw vegetables, potatoes, rice, pasta, and popcorn. They also make excellent salad dressings or can be used as the base for salad dressings. Because additional heat can change their character, these oils are used for flavoring, not for cooking.

There are two basic methods for flavoring oils. Flavoring ingredients that taste best when cooked or roasted, such as nuts and shrimp, are heated with the oil. These are called *heated oils*. Ingredients that taste better raw or lightly cooked, such as herbs, are covered with hot oil and left to sit for 30 minutes. These are called *infused oils*. Store oils in the refrigerator and use within a few days.

Heated Oils

When you use the heating method to flavor oil, the saucepan should be placed over low heat. Cook the ingredients just enough to extract the flavor, then remove the pan from the heat, put the oil into a separate container, and let it cool. Oil retains heat for some time and will continue to cook even after it has been taken off the burner. Remove from the heat before the ingredients have been completely cooked and allow the hot oil to finish the cooking. Do not overcook. You may strain the flavoring ingredients and separate them from the oil before using, or eat them along with the oil. If they are not overcooked, the flavoring ingredients usually add to the flavor and enjoyment of the oil. When making these oils, use an equal amount of coconut oil and flavoring ingredient. For example, if you have ¼ cup flavoring ingredient, cook it in ¼ cup oil. The flavored oils below use the heating method.

Toasted Coconut Oil

TOASTING DRIED COCONUT in coconut oil gives the oil a wonderful flavor. This oil makes an excellent spread in place of butter. Sauté the coconut until it is lightly browned. Remove from the heat and cool. You can use any type of dried coconut: grated, shredded, or flaked. Keep the coconut in the oil when you use it.

Sesame Seed Oil

THIS OIL MAKES a great-tasting topping on vegetables and salad dressing. Sauté the sesame seeds until they are lightly browned. Do not overcook. Keep in mind that the oil remains hot even after the pan is removed from the heat, so the sesame seeds will continue to cook for a few minutes. Keep the seeds in the oil when used.

Almond Oil

IF YOU LIKE ALMONDS, you'll love this oil. Crush or finely chop almonds and toast them in coconut oil until lightly browned. Keep the almonds in the oil when used.

Garlic Oil

THIS LIGHTLY FLAVORED oil will give foods just enough garlic flavor to waken your taste buds. Dice garlic and sauté it in coconut oil until lightly browned. Remove the garlic and use just the oil.

Onion Oil

THIS OIL will give food a hint of onion flavor. Try it on popcorn or bread. It tastes great with vegetables. Chop onion and sauté it until tender and lightly browned. Use the oil with or without the onion bits.

Shrimp Oil

DICE THE SHRIMP and cook it in hot coconut oil for only a couple of minutes. Shrimp cooks quickly; avoid overcooking. Keep the shrimp in the oil when used. This makes an excellent salad dressing or topping on vegetables. You can spruce it up by adding a little lemon juice, salt, and pepper.

Infused Oils

With the infusion method, oil is heated in a saucepan until hot. Remove the pan from the heat, add the flavoring ingredients, pour the oil into a separate container, and let it sit for about 30 minutes to allow the flavor to infuse or migrate into the oil. Always add the flavoring ingredients to the pan before pouring the oil into a separate container to avoid splattering. Strain or remove the flavoring ingredients before using the oil. When making these oils, use equal amounts of coconut oil and flavoring ingredient unless otherwise directed. So if you have ¼ cup of a flavoring ingredient, mix in ¼ cup of coconut oil. The flavored oils below use the infusion method.

Lemon Oil

LEMON GIVES MANY FOODS a welcome boost in flavor. This oil has a mild lemon flavor that will add just enough flavor to perk up your taste buds. Use finely chopped lemon peel, not the fruit. Serve with fish, asparagus, artichokes, or broccoli.

Orange Oil

LIKE LEMON, the flavor of orange can add dimension to foods. Use finely chopped or grated orange peel.

Ginger Oil

GINGER IS A WONDERFUL SPICE that can be used in main dishes, desserts, and beverages. Use finely diced fresh ginger. Remove the ginger before using the oil.

Red Pepper Oil

IF YOU WANT to add some spice to a dish, this oil can do the job. But watch out, this oil is hot! A little can go a long way. Infuse coconut oil with crushed red pepper flakes. You can use the oil with or without the red pepper pieces.

Herb Oil

YOU CAN GIVE coconut oil almost any type of herb flavor. Fresh, diced herbs work best, but dried herbs can also be used. Among the types of herbs you can use are dill, bay leaves, sage, lemon grass, and coriander, plus others.

Italian Herb Oil

This all-purpose herbal blend uses several different herbs. Use this oil as a dip for chips and raw vegetables, a topping on steamed vegetables, a spread on bread, a salad dressing, or a topping for popcorn.

> 3½ tablespoons (52 ml) coconut oil
> 2 tablespoons (20 g) finely diced onion
> 1 tablespoon (8 g) finely diced or crushed garlic
> ½ teaspoon ground basil
> ½ teaspoon ground oregano
> ¼ teaspoon paprika
> ¼ teaspoon salt
> ⅛ teaspoon freshly ground black pepper or cayenne pepper

IN A SMALL SAUCEPAN, heat the coconut oil over medium heat until hot. Remove the pan from the heat. In a small container, combine the onion, garlic, basil, oregano, paprika, salt, and pepper and add it to the hot oil. Pour the hot oil mixture into a separate container and let it sit for 30 minutes. Do not strain the oil before using. **MAKES ABOUT ½ CUP (120 ML)**

SOUPS AND CHOWDERS

Chicken and Dumplings ✿

4 cups (950 ml) chicken broth
½ cup (80 g) chopped onion
½ cup (50 g) chopped celery
½ cup (65 g) sliced carrot
½ cup (62 g) flour
1 can (14 ounces/400 ml) coconut milk or coconut cream
½ cup (75 g) peas
2 cups (280 g) cut-up chicken
1 teaspoon salt
¼ teaspoon freshly ground black pepper
½ teaspoon dried thyme
Dumplings (page 74)

IN A 3-QUART (3-LITER) SAUCEPAN, bring the broth to a boil over medium heat. Add the onion, celery, and carrot; reduce the heat to medium-low and simmer for 30 minutes. In a small bowl, mix the flour with the coconut milk; stir the mixture into the hot broth. Raise the heat to medium-high, bring the soup to a boil, and add the peas, chicken, salt, pepper, and thyme; reduce the heat to a simmer. Drop the dumplings into the soup, cover, and simmer for 20 minutes.   SERVES 6

Dumplings

>   1 cup (125 g) flour, plus extra to coat the dumplings
>   ½ teaspoon salt
>   1½ teaspoons baking powder
>   ½ cup (120 ml) coconut milk
>   1 large egg

IN A MEDIUM BOWL, mix together the flour, salt, and baking powder. In a separate bowl, mix together the coconut milk and egg. Combine the wet ingredients and the dry ingredients. Form the dough into 1-inch (2.5 cm) balls. Coat each one in flour and drop into the soup. Cook, covered, for 20 minutes.   MAKES ABOUT 12 DUMPLINGS

Hearty Chicken Stew ⚙

>   4 cups (950 ml) chicken broth
>   ½ large onion, chopped
>   1 rib celery, chopped
>   1 cup (100 g) green beans, cut into pieces
>   3 medium red potatoes, chopped
>   ¼ cup (31 g) flour
>   1 can (14 ounces/400 ml) coconut milk or coconut cream
>   ½ cup (75 g) peas
>   2 cups (280 g) bite-size pieces cooked chicken
>   1 teaspoon salt
>   ⅛ teaspoon freshly ground black pepper
>   ½ teaspoon ground sage

IN A 3-QUART (3-LITER) SAUCEPAN, bring the broth to a boil over medium-high heat. Add the onion, celery, green beans, and potatoes; reduce the heat to medium-low and simmer for 20 minutes. In a small bowl, mix the flour with the coconut milk; stir the mixture into the hot broth. Raise the heat to medium and bring the broth to a boil. Add the peas, chicken, salt, pepper, and sage. Reduce the heat to medium-low. Simmer and cook, covered, for 10 minutes.   SERVES 6

Cream of Asparagus Soup

1 pound (455 g) asparagus, washed, trimmed, and cut in 1-inch
(2.5-cm) pieces
½ cup (50 g) chopped celery
¼ cup (40 g) chopped onion
1 cup (235 ml) water
2 tablespoons (30 ml) extra-virgin olive oil
2 tablespoons (15 g) flour
1 can (14 ounces/400 ml) coconut milk
1¼ teaspoons salt
⅛ teaspoon freshly ground black pepper
¼ teaspoon dried tarragon

TO A LARGE SAUCEPAN, add the asparagus, celery, onion, and water. Simmer over medium-low heat for about 20 minutes, or until the vegetables are very tender. In the bowl of a blender, puree the mixture a little at a time at low speed. In a medium saucepan, heat the olive oil over medium heat; blend in the flour and cook for about 5 minutes, stirring frequently, until lightly browned. Add the coconut milk slowly, stirring until smooth. Mix in the puree, salt, pepper, and tarragon. Cook, stirring occasionally, for about 5 minutes, until the soup is hot but not boiling.   SERVES 4

Cream of Broccoli Soup

2 cups (142 g) chopped broccoli
½ cup (50 g) chopped celery
¼ cup (40 g) chopped onion
1 cup (235 ml) water
2 tablespoons (¼ stick/30 ml) salted butter or coconut oil
2 tablespoons (15 g) flour
1 can (14 ounces/400 ml) coconut milk
1¼ teaspoons salt
⅛ teaspoon freshly ground black pepper
¼ teaspoon dried basil

IN A MEDIUM SAUCEPAN, add the broccoli, celery, onion, and water. Simmer over medium-low heat for about 20 minutes, or until the vegetables are very tender. In the bowl of a blender, puree the mixture a little at a time at low speed. In a medium saucepan, melt the butter over medium heat; blend in the flour and cook, stirring frequently, for about 5 minutes, until lightly browned. Add the coconut milk slowly, stirring until smooth. Mix in the puree, salt, pepper, and basil. Cook, stirring occasionally, for about 5 minutes, until the soup is hot but not boiling.   SERVES 4

Cream of Cauliflower Soup

2 cups (200 g) chopped cauliflower

½ cup (50 g) chopped celery

¼ cup (40 g) chopped onion

1 cup (235 ml) water

2 tablespoons (¼ stick/30 ml) salted butter or coconut oil

2 tablespoons (15 g) flour

1 can (14 ounces/400 ml) coconut milk

1¼ teaspoons salt

⅛ teaspoon white pepper

¼ teaspoon curry powder

IN A MEDIUM SAUCEPAN, add the cauliflower, celery, onion, and water. Simmer over medium-low heat for about 20 minutes, or until the vegetables are very tender. In the bowl of a blender, puree the mixture a little at a time at low speed. In a medium saucepan, melt the butter over medium heat; blend in the flour and cook, stirring frequently, for about 5 minutes, until lightly browned. Add the coconut milk slowly, stirring until smooth. Mix in the puree, salt, pepper, and curry powder, stirring occasionally, until the soup is hot but not boiling.   SERVES 4

Curried Cream of Cauliflower Soup

2 tablespoons (30 ml) coconut oil

½ cup (80 g) chopped onion

1½ teaspoons (3 g) curry powder

⅛ teaspoon saffron

½ cup (62 g) chopped apple

3 cups (300 g) chopped cauliflower

2 cups (475 ml) water or chicken broth

1 teaspoon salt

⅛ teaspoon white pepper

½ cup (120 ml) coconut milk

IN A MEDIUM SAUCEPAN, heat the coconut oil over medium heat. Add the onion, curry, and saffron and sauté for 2 minutes, stirring often. Add the apple and cook for another 5 minutes. Add the cauliflower, water, salt, and pepper. Bring to a boil, reduce the heat to medium-low, and simmer for about 15 minutes, until the cauliflower is tender. Add the coconut milk and simmer for 2 minutes more. In the bowl of a blender, puree the soup at low speed until smooth. Serve hot.   SERVES 4

Cream of Artichoke Soup

2 tablespoons (30 ml) coconut oil or 2 tablespoons (¼ stick) salted butter

½ cup (50 g) chopped celery

¼ cup (40 g) chopped onion

2 cloves garlic, minced

2 tablespoons (15 g) flour

1 cup (235 ml) water

1 can (14 ounces/400 ml) coconut milk

1 can (14 ounces/525 g) artichoke hearts, drained and rinsed

1 teaspoon salt

¼ teaspoon white pepper

¼ teaspoon dried thyme

IN A MEDIUM HEAVY SAUCEPAN, heat the coconut oil over medium-low heat. Add the celery, onion, and garlic and sauté for about 8 minutes, until the vegetables are tender. Stir in the flour and cook for 2 minutes. Add the water and coconut milk, bring to a boil, reduce the heat to medium-low, and simmer for 8 to 10 minutes. In the bowl of a blender, add half of the mixture and all of the artichokes and puree at low speed; add the puree back to the pan. Add the salt, pepper, and thyme and heat, stirring, for 2 to 3 minutes. SERVES 4

Cream of Spinach Soup

1 pound (455 g) fresh spinach, washed and chopped (see Note)

1 rib celery, chopped

½ medium onion, chopped

3 cloves garlic, chopped

1¼ teaspoons salt

¾ teaspoon lemon pepper

2 cups (475 ml) water

1 can (14 ounces/400 ml) coconut milk

IN A LARGE SAUCEPAN, add the spinach, celery, onion, garlic, salt, lemon pepper, and water. Simmer over medium-low heat for about 30 minutes, or until the vegetables are very tender. Add the coconut milk. In the bowl of a blender, puree the mixture at low speed. Serve hot. SERVES 4

Note
You may use a 10-ounce (284-g) package of frozen spinach if desired.

Cream of Potato Soup

1 pound (455 g) potatoes, peeled and cut in 1-inch (2.5-cm) chunks

½ cup (50 g) chopped celery

¼ cup (40 g) chopped onion

1 cup (235 ml) water

2 tablespoons (30 ml) extra-virgin olive oil

2 tablespoons (15 g) flour

1 can (14 ounces/400 ml) coconut milk
1¼ teaspoons salt
⅛ teaspoon white pepper
¼ teaspoon dried dill

IN A LARGE SAUCEPAN, place the potatoes, celery, onion, and water. Simmer over medium-low heat for about 20 minutes, or until the vegetables are very tender. In the bowl of a blender, puree the mixture, a little at a time, at low speed. In a medium saucepan, heat the olive oil over medium heat; blend in the flour and cook, stirring frequently, for about 5 minutes, until lightly browned. Add the coconut milk slowly, stirring until smooth. Mix in the puree, salt, pepper, and dill, stirring occasionally, until the soup is hot but not boiling.   SERVES 4

Cream of Mushroom Soup

2 tablespoons (¼ stick/28 g) salted butter
1 cup (8 ounces/70 g) chopped mushrooms
¼ cup (40 g) chopped onion
2 tablespoons (16 g) cornstarch
1 cup (235 ml) water
1 can (14 ounces/400 ml) coconut milk
1 teaspoon salt
⅛ teaspoon white pepper
1 teaspoon Worcestershire sauce

IN A MEDIUM HEAVY SAUCEPAN, melt the butter over low heat. Add the mushrooms and onion and sauté for 5 to 7 minutes, until the vegetables are slightly tender. In a small bowl, blend together the cornstarch and water and add it to the saucepan; heat, stirring, for 3 to 4 minutes, until thickened. Add the coconut milk, reduce the heat to low, cover, and simmer, stirring occasionally, for 12 to 15 minutes, until the vegetables are tender. In the bowl of a blender, puree half of the mixture at low speed; return the puree to the pan. Add the salt, pepper, and Worcestershire sauce and heat, stirring, for 2 to 3 minutes, until hot.   SERVES 4

Creamy Zucchini Soup

    2 tablespoons (30 ml) coconut oil

    ½ cup (80 g) chopped onion

    2 cloves garlic, minced

    3 cups (710 g) water or chicken broth

    1 potato, chopped (about 1 cup/110 g)

    1 large carrot, sliced

    4 medium zucchini, cut in 1-inch (2.5 cm) cubes

    1 cup (235 ml) coconut milk

    1 tablespoon (2.5 g) fresh basil or 1 teaspoon dried basil

    1 teaspoon salt

    ⅛ teaspoon white pepper

IN A MEDIUM SAUCEPAN, heat the coconut oil over low heat. Add the onion and garlic and sauté for 2 minutes. Add the water, potato, carrot, and zucchini; bring to a boil, reduce the heat to medium-low, and simmer for about 15 minutes, until the vegetables are tender. Add the coconut milk, basil, salt, and pepper and simmer for 5 minutes. In the bowl of a blender, puree the soup at low speed until smooth. Serve hot.   SERVES 4

Creamy Tomato Soup

    2 tablespoons (30 ml) extra-virgin olive oil

    2 tablespoons (20 g) minced yellow onion

    2 tablespoons (15 g) flour

    ½ cup (120 ml) water

    ¾ cup (184 g) tomato sauce

    1 can (14 ounces/400 ml) coconut milk

    ½ teaspoon dried basil

    ½ teaspoon dried oregano

    1 teaspoon salt

    ⅛ teaspoon freshly ground black pepper

    ½ teaspoon garlic powder

IN A MEDIUM HEAVY SAUCEPAN, heat the olive oil over medium-low heat. Add the onion and sauté for about 6 minutes, until limp. Blend in the flour, then add the water, tomato sauce, coconut milk, basil, oregano, salt, pepper, and garlic powder. Raise the heat to medium-high and bring the soup to a boil. Reduce the heat to medium-low and simmer, covered, for 10 minutes, stirring occasionally. Serve hot.   SERVES 4

Creamy Tomato-Vegetable Soup

2 tablespoons (30 ml) extra-virgin olive oil

¼ cup (40 g) minced yellow onion

½ cup (50 g) chopped celery

½ cup (65 g) chopped carrot

2 tablespoons (15 g) flour

½ cup (120 ml) water

½ cup (75 g) peas

¾ cup (184 g) tomato sauce

1 can (14 ounces/400 ml) coconut milk

½ teaspoon dried basil

½ teaspoon dried oregano

1 teaspoon salt

⅛ teaspoon freshly ground black pepper

½ teaspoon garlic powder

IN A MEDIUM HEAVY SAUCEPAN, heat the olive oil over medium-low heat. Add the onion, celery, and carrot and sauté for about 6 minutes, until the vegetables are limp. Blend in the flour, then add the water, peas, tomato sauce, coconut milk, basil, oregano, salt, pepper, and garlic powder. Raise the heat to medium-high and bring to a boil. Reduce the heat to medium-low and simmer, covered, for 10 minutes, stirring occasionally. Serve hot.   SERVES 3 TO 4

Tomato-Shrimp Soup

2 tablespoons (30 ml) extra-virgin olive oil

2 tablespoons (20 g) minced yellow onion

2 tablespoons (15 g) flour

½ cup (120 ml) water

¾ cup (184 g) tomato sauce

1 can (14 ounces/400 ml) coconut milk

½ teaspoon dried basil

½ teaspoon dried oregano

1 teaspoon salt

⅛ teaspoon freshly ground black pepper

½ teaspoon garlic powder

½ cup (113 g) baby shrimp

IN A MEDIUM HEAVY SAUCEPAN, heat the olive oil over medium-low heat. Add the onion and sauté for about 6 minutes, until limp. Blend in the flour, then add the water, tomato sauce, coconut milk, basil, oregano, salt, pepper, garlic powder, and shrimp. Raise the heat to medium-high and bring the soup to a boil. Reduce the heat to medium-low and simmer, covered, for 10 minutes, stirring occasionally. Serve hot.   SERVES 2 TO 3

New England Clam Chowder

1½ cups (355 ml) water

½ cup (80 g) minced yellow onion

1 rib celery, chopped

2 cups (220 g) diced red potatoes

1 teaspoon salt

⅛ teaspoon white pepper

1 can (14 ounces/400 ml) coconut milk or cream

1 can (6½ or 8 ounces/182 or 224 g) minced or chopped clams, undrained

IN A MEDIUM SAUCEPAN, add the water, onion, celery, potatoes, salt, and pepper. Bring to a boil over medium-high heat. Reduce the heat to medium-low and simmer for about 20 minutes, or until the potatoes are tender. Add the coconut milk and clams, including the clam juice. Cook for about 5 minutes, until heated through.   SERVES 4

Deluxe Clam Chowder ⚙

½ cup (120 ml) water

½ cup (80 g) minced yellow onion

4 cloves garlic, minced

1 rib celery, chopped

2 cups (220 g) diced red potatoes

1 teaspoon salt

⅛ teaspoon white pepper

1 can (14 ounces/400 ml) coconut milk or coconut cream

1 can (8 ounces/224 g) minced or chopped clams, undrained

1 bottle (8 ounces/235 ml) clam juice

1 tablespoon (14 g) unsalted butter (optional)

¼ teaspoon paprika

IN A MEDIUM SAUCEPAN, add the water, onion, garlic, celery, potatoes, salt, and pepper. Bring to a boil over medium-high heat. Reduce the heat to medium-low and simmer for about 20 minutes, or until the potatoes are tender. Add the coconut milk and clams, including the clam juice, and the butter, if using. Cook for about 5 minutes, until heated through. Sprinkle the top with paprika and serve.   SERVES 4

Fish Chowder

1½ cups (355 ml) water

1 pound (455 g) fresh or frozen fish fillets

½ cup (80 g) minced yellow onion

2 cups (220 g) diced red potatoes

1 teaspoon salt

⅛ teaspoon white pepper

1 can (14 ounces/400 ml) coconut milk or coconut cream

CUT THE FISH into bite-size pieces. In a medium saucepan, add the water, fish, onion, potatoes, salt, and pepper. Bring to a boil over medium-high heat. Reduce the heat to medium-low and simmer for about 20 minutes, or until the potatoes are tender. Add the coconut milk and cook for about 5 minutes, until heated through.   SERVES 4

Shrimp Chowder

> 3 strips bacon
>
> ½ cup (80 g) minced yellow onion
>
> 1½ cups (355 ml) water
>
> 2 cups (220 g) diced red potatoes
>
> 1 teaspoon salt
>
> ⅛ teaspoon white pepper
>
> 1 can (14 ounces/400 ml) coconut milk or coconut cream
>
> 2 teaspoons fish sauce (see Note)
>
> ½ pound (226 g) fresh or frozen whole baby shrimp

IN A MEDIUM SKILLET, cook the bacon over medium-high heat until crisp. Remove the bacon and set aside, keeping the bacon drippings in the skillet. Add the onion and sauté in the bacon drippings for about 5 minutes, until tender. In a medium saucepan, bring to a boil the water, potatoes, salt, and pepper over medium-high heat. Reduce the heat to X and simmer for about 15 minutes, or until the potatoes are tender. Add the cooked onions, coconut milk, fish sauce, and shrimp. Cook for about 5 minutes, until heated through. Serve with bacon crumbled on top.   SERVES 4

Note

Fish sauce is available in the Asian section of the grocery store.

Crab Chowder

> 2 tablespoons (¼ stick/30 ml) salted butter or coconut oil
>
> 1 medium onion, chopped
>
> 2 ribs celery, chopped
>
> 2 cloves garlic, chopped
>
> 4 cups (950 ml) chicken broth
>
> 4 red potatoes, chopped
>
> 1 can (14¾ ounces/472 g) cream-style corn
>
> ½ teaspoon salt
>
> ½ teaspoon freshly ground black pepper
>
> ¼ cup (31 g) flour

1 can (14 ounces/400 ml) coconut milk

8 ounces (118 g) crabmeat

2 tablespoons (30 ml) fish sauce (see Note)

1 teaspoon dried thyme

IN A LARGE SAUCEPAN, melt the butter over medium heat. Add the onion, celery, and garlic and sauté for about 6 minutes, until tender. Add the broth, potatoes, corn, salt, and pepper. Raise the heat to medium-high and bring to a boil. Then reduce the heat to medium-low and simmer for about 20 minutes, or until the potatoes are tender. In a small bowl, mix the flour with the coconut milk. Add the mixture to the chowder, along with the crabmeat, fish sauce, and thyme. Cook, stirring frequently, for another 5 to 6 minutes, until the chowder is slightly thickened.   SERVES 4

Note

Fish sauce is available in the Asian section of the grocery store.

Corn Chowder

2 tablespoons (30 ml) coconut oil or bacon drippings

½ cup (80 g) chopped onion

½ cup (75 g) chopped bell pepper

2 tablespoons (15 g) flour

¾ cup (175 ml) water

1 can (14 ounces/400 ml) coconut milk

2 cups (330 g) frozen or canned corn

1 teaspoon salt

¼ teaspoon freshly ground black pepper

1 jar (4 ounces/96 g) pimiento

2 teaspoons fish sauce (see Note)

4 strips bacon, crisp-cooked and crumbled (optional)

IN A LARGE SAUCEPAN, heat the coconut oil over medium heat. Add the onion and bell pepper and sauté for about 5 minutes, until tender. Add the flour and cook for 3 to 4 minutes, until lightly browned. Add the water, coconut milk, corn, salt, and pepper. Raise the heat to medium-high and bring to a boil, stirring constantly. Reduce the heat to medium-low and simmer for about 10 minutes, until the vegetables are tender. In the bowl of a blender, place half of the mixture and puree at low speed; return the puree to the pan. Add the pimiento and fish sauce. Heat, stirring constantly, for 2 to 3 minutes, until hot. Serve topped with crumbled bacon if desired. SERVES 3 TO 4

Note
Fish sauce is available in the Asian section of the grocery store.

Corn and Potato Chowder

> 2 medium potatoes, chopped
> 1 medium onion, thinly sliced and separated into rings
> ½ cup (50 g) chopped celery
> 1 teaspoon salt
> ½ cup (120 ml) water
> 2 cups (512 g) whole kernel corn
> 1 can (4 ounces/96 g) pimiento
> 1 can (14 ounces/400 ml) coconut milk or coconut cream
> ¼ teaspoon dried marjoram, crushed
> ⅛ teaspoon white pepper
> 1 tablespoon (14 g) salted butter (optional)
> 5 strips bacon, crisp-cooked and crumbled (optional)

IN A LARGE SAUCEPAN, combine the potatoes, onion, celery, salt, and water. Cover and cook over medium heat for about 15 minutes, or until the vegetables are tender. Stir in the corn, pimiento, coconut milk, marjoram, and pepper. Reduce the heat to medium-low and simmer, covered, for 5 minutes. Add the butter if you like and serve topped with crumbled bacon if desired. SERVES 4

Oyster Stew ✿

> 1½ cups (355 ml) water
> ½ cup (40 g) minced yellow onion

1 rib celery, chopped

2 cups (220 g) diced potatoes

1 teaspoon salt

⅛ teaspoon white pepper

1 can (14 ounces/400 ml) coconut milk or coconut cream

1 tablespoon (14 g) salted butter

1 can (8 ounces/248 g) oysters, undrained

IN A MEDIUM SAUCEPAN, add the water, onion, celery, potatoes, salt, and pepper. Bring to a boil over medium-high heat. Reduce the heat to medium-low and simmer for about 20 minutes, or until the potatoes are tender. Add the coconut milk, butter, and oysters, including the oyster juice. Cook for about 5 minutes, until heated through. SERVES 4

Potato Soup

2 tablespoons (30 ml) coconut oil

1 small yellow onion, peeled and minced

½ cup (50 g) chopped celery

½ cup (4 ounces/35 g) chopped mushrooms

2 cups (220 g) diced peeled potatoes

2 cups (475 ml) water or chicken broth

1 teaspoon salt

1 can (14 ounces/400 ml) coconut milk or coconut cream

⅛ teaspoon white pepper

1 tablespoon (4 g) minced fresh parsley, chives, or dill

Crumbled bacon, as garnish (optional)

IN A HEAVY SAUCEPAN, heat the coconut oil over medium heat. Add the onion and celery and sauté for about 5 minutes, until the vegetables are limp. Add the mushrooms, potatoes, water, and salt. Reduce the heat to medium-low. Cover the pan and simmer for 10 to 15 minutes, until the potatoes are nearly tender. Add the coconut milk and pepper and simmer uncovered, stirring occasionally, for 3 to 5 minutes, until the potatoes are tender. Sprinkle with the parsley and serve. Crumbled bacon also goes well as a garnish. SERVES 4

Potato and Sausage Soup

1 pound (455 g) sausage

¼ cup (20 g) chopped onion

½ cup (75 g) chopped green bell pepper

3 tablespoons (23 g) flour

3 cups (710 ml) water

1 can (14 ounces/400 ml) coconut milk

3 red potatoes, chopped

1 teaspoon salt

⅛ teaspoon freshly ground black pepper

1 teaspoon ground sage

IN A HEAVY SAUCEPAN, add the sausage, onion, and bell pepper. Cook over medium heat for about 5 minutes, until the meat is browned and the vegetables are tender. Stir in the flour and cook for 1 minute. Add the water, coconut milk, potatoes, salt, and pepper and bring to a boil. Reduce the heat to medium-low and simmer for about 20 minutes, or until the potatoes are tender. Add the sage and simmer for 5 minutes more.   SERVES 6

Ham and Potato Soup

4 cups (950 ml) water

1 meaty ham bone (1½ pounds/680 g)

½ medium onion, chopped

1 rib celery, chopped

1 carrot, chopped

3 red potatoes, chopped

1 can (14 ounces/400 ml) coconut milk

1 teaspoon salt

⅛ teaspoon freshly ground black pepper

¼ teaspoon dried marjoram

IN A LARGE, heavy saucepan, combine the water, ham bone, onion, celery, and carrot. Bring to a boil over medium-high heat. Cover, reduce the heat to medium-low, and simmer for 2 hours. Remove the ham bone from the soup;

cut off the meat and dice it. Return the meat to the soup. Add the potatoes, coconut milk, salt, pepper, and marjoram. Simmer, covered, for about 20 minutes, or until the potatoes are tender.   SERVES 6

Chicken and Rice Stew

3 tablespoons (45 ml) coconut oil

1 small yellow onion, minced

1 medium carrot, peeled and finely diced

1 rib celery, finely diced

½ green bell pepper, cored, seeded, and minced

¼ cup (31 g) flour

1 tablespoon (6 g) curry powder

¼ teaspoon ground nutmeg

1 teaspoon ground cloves

1 teaspoon dried parsley

3 cups (710 ml) chicken broth

1 teaspoon salt

⅛ teaspoon freshly ground black pepper

1 cup (180 g) chopped fresh tomatoes

1 cup (140 g) cooked diced chicken

1 can (14 ounces/400 ml) coconut milk

1 cup (165 g) cooked rice

IN A LARGE SAUCEPAN, heat the coconut oil over medium heat. Add the onion, carrot, celery, and bell pepper and cook for 8 to 10 minutes, until the onion is slightly golden. Stir in the flour, curry powder, and nutmeg; add the cloves, parsley, broth, salt, pepper, and tomatoes. Reduce the heat to medium-low. Cover and simmer for 30 minutes. Remove the pan from the heat. Strain the broth, separating the vegetables from the liquid. In the bowl of a blender, puree the vegetables at low speed. Stir the puree into the broth. Add the chicken and coconut milk; cook over medium heat, stirring occasionally, for 5 to 6 minutes, until hot. Add the cooked rice and continue to cook until heated through.   SERVES 6

Red Lentil Soup

2 tablespoons (30 ml) coconut oil

1 large onion, chopped

3 medium carrots, peeled and chopped

4 cups (950 ml) water

1 can (14 ounces/400 ml) coconut milk

1 cup (192 g) red lentils

3 cloves garlic, chopped

1 bay leaf

2 teaspoons salt

¼ teaspoon ground ginger

1 tablespoon (6 g) curry powder

½ cup (8 g) chopped fresh cilantro

IN A LARGE SAUCEPAN, heat the coconut oil over medium heat. Add the onion and carrots and cook, stirring frequently, for about 10 minutes, until the vegetables start to brown. Add the water, coconut milk, lentils, garlic, bay leaf, salt, ginger, and curry powder. Cover and bring to a boil. Reduce the heat to medium-low and simmer, partially covered, stirring occasionally, for 35 to 40 minutes, or until the lentils are tender. Add the cilantro and cook for 3 minutes more. Remove the bay leaf and discard. In the bowl of a blender, puree the soup in batches until velvety smooth. Serve hot.   SERVES 5 TO 6

Creamy Cheese and Broccoli Soup

4 cups (950 ml) chicken broth

½ medium onion, chopped

1 rib celery, chopped

½ head of broccoli, chopped

1 teaspoon salt

⅛ teaspoon freshly ground black pepper

½ teaspoon dried basil

2 cups (475 ml) Creamy Cheese Sauce (page 63)

IN A 3-QUART SAUCEPAN, bring the broth to a boil over medium-high heat. Add the onion, celery, broccoli, salt, pepper, and basil. Reduce the heat to medium-low and simmer for about 30 minutes, until the vegetables are very tender. Remove the pan from the heat. In the bowl of a blender, puree the soup until smooth. Return the puree to the pan and add the Creamy Cheese Sauce. Over low to medium-low heat, stir the cheese sauce into the soup until well blended and hot. Remove from the heat and serve.

SERVES 4

Cheese and Potato Soup

> 2 tablespoons (30 ml) coconut oil
>
> 1 small yellow onion, minced
>
> 1 rib celery, chopped
>
> ½ cup (4 ounces/35 g) chopped fresh mushrooms
>
> 2 potatoes, chopped
>
> 2 cups (475 ml) water
>
> 2 cups (475 ml) chicken broth
>
> 1 teaspoon salt
>
> ¼ teaspoon freshly ground black pepper
>
> 1 cup (140 g) bite-size pieces of cooked chicken
>
> 1 teaspoon minced dill
>
> 3 cups (710 ml) Creamy Cheese Sauce (page 63)

IN A HEAVY SAUCEPAN, heat the coconut oil over medium heat. Add the onion and celery and sauté for about 5 minutes, until limp. Add the mushrooms, potatoes, water, broth, salt, and pepper. Cover, reduce the heat to medium-low, and simmer for about 15 minutes, or until the potatoes are tender. Mix in the chicken, dill, and Creamy Cheddar Cheese Sauce and simmer, stirring frequently, for 5 minutes. Remove from the heat and serve.

SERVES 4

Beefy Cheese Soup 🌼

> 1 tablespoon (15 ml) coconut oil
>
> 1 pound (455 g) ground beef
>
> 1 medium onion, chopped
>
> 4 cups (950 ml) water

1 cup (260 g) salsa

2 potatoes, chopped

1½ cups (150 g) chopped green beans

2 cups (475 ml) Creamy Cheese Sauce (page 63)

1½ teaspoons salt

¼ teaspoon freshly ground black pepper

½ teaspoon dried thyme

IN A LARGE SAUCEPAN, heat the coconut oil over medium heat. Add the ground beef and onion and cook for about 7 minutes, until the onion is tender and the beef is browned. Add the water, salsa, potatoes, and green beans. Bring to a boil, then reduce the heat to medium-low. Cover and simmer for about 15 minutes, or until the potatoes are tender. Stir in the Creamy Cheese Sauce, salt, pepper, and thyme. Simmer for 5 minutes more and serve.   SERVES 4

Tamale Soup ⚙

1 tablespoon (15 ml) coconut oil

1 pound (455 g) ground beef

1 small onion, chopped

½ bell pepper, seeded and chopped

4 cups (950 ml) water

3 tablespoons (23 g) flour

1 cup (235 ml) Creamy Cheese Sauce (page 63)

1 cup (171 g) cooked pinto beans

½ cup (83 g) whole kernel corn

1 can (8 ounces/245 g) tomato sauce

½ cup (130 g) salsa

1 teaspoon chili powder

1 teaspoon ground cumin

1 teaspoon salt

Corn Bread Dumplings (page 63)

IN A LARGE SAUCEPAN, heat the coconut oil over medium heat. Add the ground beef, onion, and bell pepper and sauté until the vegetables are tender and the meat is browned. In a small bowl, mix together the water and flour and pour it into the saucepan. Add the Creamy Cheese Sauce, pinto beans, corn, tomato sauce, salsa, chili powder, cumin, and salt. Bring to a boil, then reduce the heat to medium-low. Simmer, stirring frequently, for 10 minutes. Drop the Corn Bread Dumplings into the hot soup. Cover and simmer for 20 minutes. Serve hot with the dumplings.   SERVES 6

Corn Bread Dumplings

½ cup (120 ml) coconut milk

1 large egg

½ cup (70 g) cornmeal

¼ cup (31 g) flour, plus more for coating the dumplings

1 teaspoon baking powder

1 teaspoon sugar

¼ teaspoon salt

IN A SMALL BOWL, combine the coconut milk and egg; mix thoroughly. In a separate medium bowl, mix together the cornmeal, flour, baking powder, sugar, and salt. Add the dry ingredients to the wet ingredients, mixing just until moistened. Form the dough into 1-inch (25-mm) balls and roll in flour to coat the surface. Drop the dumplings into the hot soup.
MAKES 12 DUMPLINGS

Butternut Soup

This is a slightly sweet vegetarian soup that even meat eaters would enjoy.

2 tablespoons (30 ml) coconut oil

1 medium onion, chopped

1 carrot, sliced

1 rib celery, chopped

½ butternut squash, peeled and chopped

1 large tart apple, peeled, cored, and chopped

1 tablespoon (5.5 g) ground ginger

2 cups (475 ml) water

1 can (14 ounces/400 ml) coconut milk

½ teaspoon salt

IN A LARGE SAUCEPAN, heat the coconut oil over medium heat. Add the onion, carrot, and celery and sauté for about 7 minutes, until the vegetables are tender. Add the butternut squash, apple, ginger, water, coconut milk, and salt. Bring to a boil. Reduce the heat to medium-low, cover, and simmer for about 40 minutes, or until all of the vegetables are very soft. Remove the pan from the heat. In the bowl of a blender, puree the soup at low speed. Serve hot.   SERVES 3

Thai Chicken and Shrimp Soup

> 3 cups (710 ml) water or chicken broth
> 1 cup (235 ml) bottled clam juice
> 1 tablespoon (15 ml) fish sauce
> 2 cloves garlic, diced
> 1 teaspoon ground ginger
> ½ teaspoon red curry paste
> 1 (8-ounce/70-g) package fresh mushrooms, sliced
> 2 to 3 chicken breasts, cut into bite-size pieces
> ½ cup (4 ounces/75 g) snow peas
> ½ pound (226 g) shrimp, peeled and deveined
> 1 can (14 ounces/400 ml) coconut milk or coconut cream
> 3 scallions (white and green parts), sliced
> 2 tablespoons (2 g) chopped fresh cilantro

IN A LARGE SAUCEPAN, combine the water, clam juice, fish sauce, garlic, ginger, curry paste, mushrooms, chicken, and snow peas. Bring to a boil over medium-high heat, then reduce the heat to medium-low and simmer for 10 minutes. Add the shrimp and coconut milk and simmer for 5 minutes. Add the scallions and cilantro and cook for 1 minute more. Serve hot.

SERVES 6

MAIN DISHES

Chicken Stir-Fry

¼ cup (60 ml) coconut oil

1 medium onion, chopped

3 cloves garlic, chopped

½ bell pepper, chopped

½ head of broccoli, sliced

1 pound (455 g) chicken, cut into bite-size pieces

1 cup (8 ounces/70 g) sliced mushrooms

1 can (8½ ounces/193 g) bamboo shoots, drained

1 teaspoon ground ginger

1 teaspoon salt

3 tablespoons (24 g) cornstarch

2½ cups (595 ml) chicken broth or water

¼ cup (60 ml) soy sauce or tamari sauce

Fried Wonton Skins (page 96)

IN A LARGE SKILLET, heat the coconut oil over medium heat. Add the onion, garlic, bell pepper, and broccoli and sauté until slightly tender. Add the chicken, mushrooms, bamboo shoots, ginger, and salt. Cover and cook, stirring occasionally, for about 5 minutes, until the chicken turns white and is cooked through. In a small bowl, blend the cornstarch into the broth and add the mixture to the skillet, stirring constantly, for about 4 minutes, until the sauce is thick and bubbly. Remove the skillet from the heat. Stir in the soy sauce. Serve topped with fried wonton skins broken into bite-size pieces. SERVES 2

Fried Wonton Skins

IN A SMALL SKILLET, add coconut oil to a depth of about ¼ inch (6 mm). Heat the oil over medium heat. Put the wonton skins in the oil one at a time and cook for about 30 seconds, then turn and cook the other side for about 1 minute, or until golden brown. Remove the wonton skins from the oil and place on a paper towel–lined plate to drain. Repeat until you have 6 to 12 cooked wonton skins. Break each wonton skin into several pieces and use as a garnish.   MAKES 6 TO 12 FRIED WONTON SKINS

BEEF STIR-FRY

Make the Chicken Stir-Fry (page 95) according to the instructions, but delete the chicken and add boneless top loin steak or tenderloin, cut into bite-size pieces. SERVES 2

Almond Chicken Stir-Fry

¼ cup (60 ml) coconut oil

1 medium onion, chopped

3 cloves garlic, chopped

1 rib celery, chopped

1 bell pepper, chopped

½ cup (55 g) slivered or chopped almonds

1 pound (455 g) uncooked chicken, cut into bite-size pieces

1 cup (8 ounces/70 g) sliced fresh mushrooms

2 cups (100 g) mung bean sprouts

2 tablespoons (16 g) cornstarch

1 cup (235 ml) chicken broth or water

1 teaspoon salt

¼ cup (60 ml) soy sauce or tamari sauce

Fried Wonton Skins (page 96)

IN A LARGE SKILLET, heat the coconut oil over medium heat. Add the onion, garlic, celery, and bell pepper and sauté until the vegetables are tender. Add the almonds, chicken, and mushrooms. Cover and cook, stirring occasionally, for 4 to 5 minutes, until the chicken turns white and is cooked through. Add the bean sprouts and cook for 4 to 5 minutes more, until the vegetables are tender. In a small bowl, mix the cornstarch with the broth and add the mixture to the skillet, stirring constantly, for about 4 minutes, until thick and bubbly. Remove the skillet from the heat. Stir in the salt and soy sauce. Serve topped with fried wonton skins broken into bite-size pieces. SERVES 2

Chicken Potpie ⚙

Potpies make great meals for lunch or dinner. If you make several at a time, you can refrigerate cooked pies for a quick and easy lunch. Just reheat for a few minutes and serve. They actually taste better the second day. Uncooked pies can be frozen and used at any time for an easy, ready-to-cook and -eat meal. Frozen pies should be removed from the freezer and be allowed to thaw for at least 1 hour before baking. You can also thaw frozen pies by putting them in the refrigerator overnight.

> 2¾ cups (475 ml) water
> 1 can (14 ounces/400 ml) coconut milk
> ½ cup (80 g) chopped onion
> ½ cup (50 g) chopped celery
> ½ cup (75 g) peas
> 1 cup (110 g) chopped potatoes
> 1 teaspoon dried thyme
> 1 teaspoon salt
> ¼ teaspoon freshly ground black pepper
> 2 cups (280 g) cut-up cooked chicken
> 3 tablespoons (24 g) cornstarch
> 4 or 5 Tart Pastry Shells (page 195)

PREHEAT THE OVEN TO 400°F (200°C). In a large saucepan, add 2 cups of the water and the coconut milk and bring to a boil over medium-high heat. Add the onion, celery, peas, potatoes, thyme, salt, and pepper. Reduce the heat to medium-low and simmer, covered, for 15 minutes. Add the chicken. In a small bowl, mix the cornstarch with the remaining ¾ cup of water and add to the hot mixture, stirring constantly, for about 4 minutes, until thick and bubbly, then remove the pan from the heat.

Place the unbaked pastry shells on a baking sheet. Fill the shells with the hot mixture. Add a top crust to the pastry shells. Cut a few slits on top of the crusts. Bake for 30 to 35 minutes, until the crust is golden brown.

SERVES 2

Vegetable-Beef Potpie ❁

This is a good way to use leftover beef. You may also use fresh beef or hamburger if you like.

> 4¾ cups (1,121 ml) cold water
> 2 cups (450 g) chopped beef
> ½ cup (80 g) chopped onion
> 1 medium carrot, sliced
> ½ cup (75 g) peas
> 1 potato, chopped
> 1 teaspoon salt
> ⅛ teaspoon freshly ground black pepper
> 1 teaspoon marjoram
> ½ teaspoon paprika
> 3 tablespoons (24 g) cornstarch
> 4 or 5 Tart Pastry Shells (page 195)

PREHEAT THE OVEN TO 400°F (200°C). In a large saucepan, bring 4 cups of the water to a boil over medium-high heat. Add the meat, onion, carrot, peas, potato, salt, pepper, marjoram, and paprika. Reduce the heat to medium-low and simmer for 15 minutes. In a small bowl, mix the cornstarch with the remaining ¾ cup cold water and stir. Slowly add to the hot mixture, stirring constantly, for about 4 minutes, until thick and bubbly; remove from the heat.

Place the unbaked pastry shells on a baking sheet. Fill the shells with the hot mixture. Add a top crust to the pastry shells. Cut a few slits on top

of the crusts. Bake for 30 to 35 minutes, until the crust is golden brown.
SERVES 2

Creamy Shrimp Linguine ⚙

Linguine is pasta that is long, narrow, and flat. You can substitute spaghetti
or any other pasta of your choice in this recipe.

> 8 ounces (28 g) linguine
> 3 tablespoons (45 ml) coconut oil
> 1 medium onion, chopped
> 4 cloves garlic, chopped
> 1 cup (8 ounces/70 g) sliced fresh mushrooms
> ½ pound (226 g) shrimp, peeled, deveined, and tails removed
> 1½ cups (355 ml) Creamy Cheese Sauce (page 63)
> 2 teaspoons fish sauce (see Note)
> Fresh parsley, for garnish

PREPARE THE PASTA according to the package directions. To make the
sauce: In a large saucepan, heat the coconut oil over medium heat. Add
the onion and garlic and sauté for about 6 minutes, until tender. Add the
mushrooms and shrimp and cook for 7 to 8 minutes, until the shrimp is
pink. Stir in the Creamy Cheese Sauce, reduce the heat to low, and simmer
for 2 to 3 minutes, until hot. Stir in the fish sauce, then remove the pan from
the heat. Serve the sauce over the hot pasta. Garnish with fresh parsley.
SERVES 2 TO 3

Note
Fish sauce is available in the Asian section of the grocery store. You may substitute tamari
sauce for fish sauce if you desire.

Chicken Linguine

MAKE THE CREAMY SHRIMP LINGUINE (above) but replace the shrimp with
½ pound (226 g) of chicken cut into bite-size pieces, delete the fish sauce,
and add 1 teaspoon of salt, ¼ teaspoon of freshly ground pepper, and
½ teaspoon of basil.

Lasagna

> Coconut oil or extra-virgin olive oil, for greasing the baking pan
>
> 1 pound (455 g) ground beef
>
> 1 onion, chopped
>
> 6 cloves garlic, diced
>
> 2 cans (8 ounces/245 g each) tomato sauce
>
> 1 can (6 ounces/75 g) black olives
>
> 1½ teaspoons (1 g) dried basil
>
> 1½ teaspoons (2 g) dried oregano
>
> 1½ teaspoons salt
>
> ⅛ teaspoon freshly ground black pepper
>
> 1 package (8 or 10 ounces/38 or 48 g) lasagna noodles
>
> 2 cups (475 ml) Thick Cheddar Cheese Sauce (page 63)
>
> 2 cups (230 g) shredded mozzarella cheese
>
> Croutons (below)

PREHEAT THE OVEN TO 375°F (190°C). Coat the bottom of a 13 x 9 x 2-inch (33 x 23 x 5-cm) baking pan with coconut oil. In a medium skillet, cook the meat, onion, and garlic over medium heat for about 10 minutes, until the meat is browned and the vegetables are tender. Add the tomato sauce, olives, basil, oregano, salt, and pepper. Reduce the heat to low and simmer for 5 minutes. Cook the noodles in boiling salted water until al dente; drain and rinse. Layer one-third of the noodles on the bottom of the prepared baking pan; add the meat mixture on top of the noodles. Layer another one-third of the noodles on top of the meat mixture; spread the Thick Cheddar Cheese Sauce on top of the noodles. Layer the remaining one-third of the noodles over the cheddar cheese, followed by the mozzarella cheese. Top with croutons (recipe below). Bake for 35 minutes. Let stand for 10 minutes before serving.   SERVES 2 TO 3

Croutons

LIGHTLY TOAST 4 SLICES of bread in a toaster. Spread the toast with butter and sprinkle with garlic powder. Cut into small cubes.

MAKES ABOUT 1 CUP

Chicken Amandine

>   6 ounces (28 g) noodles
>   2 tablespoons (30 ml) coconut oil
>   ½ onion, chopped
>   3 chicken breasts, cut into bite-size pieces
>   ½ cup (55 g) slivered almonds
>   ½ teaspoon salt
>   1 cup (235 ml) Creamy Cheese Sauce (page 63)

PREHEAT THE OVEN TO 350°F (180°C). Prepare the pasta according to the package directions. In a large skillet, heat the coconut oil over medium heat. Add the onion and sauté for about 6 minutes, until tender. Add the chicken and cook until the color changes and the chicken is cooked through. Remove the skillet from the heat. Bake the almonds on a rimmed baking sheet in the oven for about 10 minutes, or until lightly browned. Add the toasted almonds, salt, and Creamy Cheese Sauce to the chicken mixture and mix. Add the cooked noodles and mix until the noodles are thoroughly coated with sauce.   SERVES 2

Beef Stroganoff

>   2 teaspoons coconut oil
>   1 pound (455 g) beef sirloin, cut into 4-inch-thick (10 cm-thick) strips
>   1 medium onion, chopped
>   4 cloves garlic, minced
>   ½ cup (4 ounces/35 g) fresh mushrooms
>   ¼ cup (60 ml) tomato sauce
>   1½ cups (355 ml) Creamy Cheese Sauce (page 63)
>   ½ teaspoon salt
>   ⅛ teaspoon freshly ground black pepper
>   1 cup (230 g) plain yogurt or sour cream
>   8 ounces (38 g) noodles of choice

IN A LARGE SKILLET, heat the coconut oil over medium heat. Add the sirloin strips and lightly brown both sides. Add the onion, garlic, and mushrooms and cook for about 8 minutes, until the vegetables are tender. Stir in the tomato sauce, Creamy Cheese Sauce, salt, and pepper. Remove from the heat and blend in the yogurt. Serve over hot noodles.   SERVES 2

Tuna Noodle Casserole

6 ounces (28 g) pasta of choice

2 tablespoons (30 ml) coconut oil

½ medium onion, chopped

½ cup (4 ounces/35 g) mushrooms, sliced

½ cup (75 g) peas

1 jar (2 ounces/48 g) pimiento

1 teaspoon salt

⅛ teaspoon freshly ground black pepper

1 can (6 ounces/170 g) tuna

1½ cups (355 ml) Creamy Cheese Sauce (page 63)

3 slices bread

2 tablespoons (¼ stick/28 g) salted butter

Garlic powder

PREHEAT THE OVEN TO 425°F (220°C). Cook the pasta according to the package directions. In a large skillet, heat the coconut oil over medium heat. Add the onion and sauté for about 6 minutes, until tender. Add the mushrooms, peas, pimiento, salt, and pepper. Cover and cook, stirring occasionally, for about 5 minutes, until the vegetables are tender. In a medium bowl, mix together the tuna, the vegetables, cooked pasta, and Creamy Cheese Sauce and pour into a 9 x 9 x 2-inch (23 x 23 x 5-cm) baking pan. Lightly toast the bread slices. Butter the bread and sprinkle with garlic powder. Break the bread into small pieces and sprinkle on top of the casserole. Bake for 15 to 20 minutes, or until the bread crumbs are browned.   SERVES 2

Orange-Coconut Chicken

 1 large egg, slightly beaten

 ¼ cup (60 ml) freshly squeezed orange juice

 1 cup (85 g) flaked coconut

 ⅓ cup (40 g) flour or dry bread crumbs

 1 teaspoon salt

 ½ teaspoon paprika

 1 teaspoon lemon pepper

 1 3-pound (1.4 kg) chicken, cut into serving-size pieces

PREHEAT THE OVEN TO 400°F (200°C). In a small bowl, mix together the egg and orange juice. In a separate medium bowl, mix together the coconut, flour, salt, paprika, and lemon pepper. Dip the chicken pieces into the orange juice mixture and then into the coconut mixture. Place the chicken, skin side down, in a baking pan large enough to accommodate all of the chicken in a single layer. Bake for 60 minutes.   SERVES 4 TO 6

Sesame Chicken ⚙

 2 tablespoons (18 g) sesame seeds

 ¼ cup (60 ml) coconut oil

 ¾ cup (120 g) diced onion

 3 cloves garlic, diced

 4 to 6 chicken breasts, cut into bite-size pieces

 ⅓ cup (50 g) peas

 ½ teaspoon ground ginger

 1 teaspoon crushed red pepper

 ½ teaspoon salt

 3 tablespoons (45 ml) tamari sauce

 6 to 8 ounces (28 to 38 g) noodles

IN A LARGE SKILLET, toast the sesame seeds in the coconut oil over medium heat for about 4 minutes, until lightly browned. Add the onion and garlic and cook, stirring occasionally, for about 6 minutes, until tender. Add the chicken, peas, ginger, red pepper, and salt. Bring to a boil, then reduce the heat to medium-low, cover, and simmer, stirring occasionally, for 10 minutes. Stir in the tamari sauce and remove the skillet from the heat. Cook the noodles according to the package directions. Drain and stir into the chicken mixture, thoroughly coating the noodles with sauce.   SERVES 4 TO 6

Almond Chicken with Noodles

½ cup (55 g) slivered almonds

¼ cup (60 ml) coconut oil

1 onion, diced

4 cloves garlic, diced

4 to 6 chicken breasts, cut into bite-size pieces

½ head of broccoli, cut into bite-size pieces

1½ cups (355 ml) coconut milk

½ teaspoon ground ginger

½ teaspoon salt

3 tablespoons (45 ml) tamari sauce

6 to 8 ounces (28 to 38 g) noodles

IN A LARGE SKILLET, toast the almonds in the coconut oil over medium heat for about 4 minutes, until lightly browned. Add the onion and garlic and cook, stirring occasionally, for about 6 minutes, until tender. Add the chicken, broccoli, coconut milk, ginger, and salt. Bring to a boil, then reduce the heat to medium-low, cover, and simmer, stirring occasionally, for 10 minutes. Stir in the tamari sauce and remove the skillet from the heat. Cook the noodles according to the package directions. Drain and stir into the chicken mixture, thoroughly coating the noodles with sauce.   SERVES 4 TO 6

Shrimp and Pasta

Freshly squeezed juice of 1 lemon

1 onion, finely chopped

½ bell pepper, seeded and finely chopped

4 cloves garlic, diced

1 tablespoon (15 ml) white vinegar

½ teaspoon salt

1 pound (455 g) fresh shrimp, shelled and deveined

1 can (14 ounces/400 ml) coconut milk

¼ cup (31 g) flour

2 tablespoons (32 g) tomato paste or ¼ cup (61 g) tomato sauce

⅛ teaspoon cayenne pepper

1 tablespoon (1 g) chopped fresh cilantro

6 ounces (28 g) pasta

IN A MEDIUM BOWL, combine the lemon juice, onion, bell pepper, garlic, vinegar, and salt to make a marinade. Add the shrimp and marinate for 30 minutes. In a large saucepan, blend together the coconut milk and flour. Add the marinade and shrimp mixture, along with the tomato paste and cayenne. Cook over low heat, stirring frequently, for about 10 minutes, or until the vegetables are cooked and the mixture is slightly thickened. Add the cilantro, cook for 1 to 2 minutes, and remove from the heat. Serve over a bed of hot pasta. **MAKES ABOUT 3 SERVINGS**

Salmon in Coconut Cream Sauce ✿

1 to 1½ pounds (455 to 680 g) salmon fillets

1 can (14 ounces/400 ml) coconut milk

1 tablespoon (8 g) cornstarch

1 teaspoon curry powder

⅛ teaspoon salt

⅛ teaspoon white pepper

½ cup (90 g) chopped fresh tomato

¼ cup (4 g) chopped fresh cilantro

PREHEAT THE OVEN TO 350°F (180°C). Put the salmon in a 11 x 7 x 1.5-inch/28 x 18 x 4-cm casserole dish. In a small bowl, blend together the coconut milk, cornstarch, curry powder, salt, and pepper and pour the sauce over the salmon. Bake for 1 hour. Serve the salmon with the coconut cream sauce garnished with fresh tomato and cilantro. This goes well with a little of the sauce poured on top of a side dish of vegetables such as broccoli, green beans, or peas. **SERVES 4**

Fried Sole with Coconut

¼ cup (60 ml) coconut milk

2 tablespoons (30 ml) freshly squeezed lime juice

1 teaspoon soy sauce

4 to 6 (4-ounce/130-g) sole fillets

¼ cup (31 g) flour

½ teaspoon ground coriander

½ teaspoon ground cumin

⅛ teaspoon cayenne pepper

½ teaspoon salt

1 tablespoon (15 ml) coconut oil

¼ cup (21 g) shredded coconut, toasted

2 tablespoons (2 g) minced fresh cilantro

1 mango, pitted and sliced

Lime wedges, for serving

IN A SMALL BOWL, mix the coconut milk, lime juice, and soy sauce. Arrange the fish fillets in a large, shallow dish. Pour the coconut milk mixture over the fish and let sit for 1 hour. Mix together the flour, coriander, cumin, cayenne, and salt. Remove the fish from the coconut milk and pat dry. Dredge the fillets in the flour mixture, shaking off any excess. In a large skillet, heat the coconut oil over medium heat. Cook the fish in the skillet, turning after about 4 minutes; cook the other side the same amount of time. Remove the fish from the heat and place on a serving dish. Garnish with the toasted coconut and cilantro. Serve with sliced mango and lime wedges.   SERVES 4

Catfish in Coconut Sauce

2 teaspoons (30 ml) coconut oil

1 pound (455 g) catfish (2 to 3 fillets)

1 medium onion, sliced

4 cloves garlic, minced

2 medium carrots, sliced

1 cup (100 g) green beans

1½ cups (355 ml) coconut milk

½ teaspoon ground ginger

1 teaspoon salt

¼ teaspoon freshly ground black pepper

2 tablespoons (30 ml) freshly squeezed lemon juice

⅓ cup (75 g) chopped cashews, for garnish

IN A LARGE SKILLET, heat the coconut oil over medium heat. Add the fish and lightly sauté both sides in the oil. Add the onion, garlic, carrots, and green beans and cook for about 5 minutes, until crisp and tender. Add the coconut milk, ginger, salt, and pepper. Cover, reduce the heat to medium-low, and simmer for about 10 minutes, until the vegetables are tender and the flavors are blended. Add the lemon juice. Remove the skillet from the heat. Garnish the fish with the cashews before serving.   SERVES 2 TO 3

Chicken Rice Casserole ⚙

¾ cup (142 g) brown rice

2¼ cups (530 ml) water

2 tablespoons (30 ml) coconut oil

½ medium onion, chopped

1 rib celery, chopped

½ bell pepper, seeded and chopped

3 to 4 chicken breasts, cut into bite-size pieces (see Note)

⅓ cup (42 g) flour

1½ teaspoons salt

⅛ teaspoon freshly ground black pepper

½ cup (4 ounces/35 g) chopped fresh mushrooms

1 can (4 ounces/96 g) pimiento

1 cup (235 ml) chicken broth

1 cup (235 ml) coconut milk

1 cup (155 g) shredded cheese (cheddar, Swiss, or Monterey)

Cayenne pepper (optional)

IN A 1-QUART SAUCEPAN, combine the rice and water. Allow the rice to soak for at least 4 hours or overnight. To cook the rice, cover and simmer over medium-low heat for 45 minutes, or until the water is absorbed and the rice is tender. Set aside. Preheat the oven to 350°F (180°C). In a large skillet, heat the coconut oil over medium heat. Add the onion, celery, and bell pepper and sauté for about 6 minutes, until tender. Add the chicken and blend in the flour, salt, and pepper. Add the mushrooms, pimiento, broth, and coconut milk. Bring to a boil, then reduce the heat to low and simmer, stirring frequently. Cook until the mixture thickens slightly and the chicken is cooked. Combine the chicken mixture with the rice and pour into a 11 x 7 x 1.5-inch/28 x 18 x 4-cm baking pan. Top with the shredded cheese and a little cayenne if desired. Cook uncovered in the oven for 35 minutes.

SERVES 3

Note

You may substitute 1 6-ounce (170 g) can of tuna for the chicken if you desire.

Chicken à La King ❁

2 tablespoons (30 ml) coconut oil

½ onion, chopped

½ green pepper, seeded and chopped

⅓ cup (42 g) flour

1 teaspoon salt

¼ teaspoon freshly ground black pepper

1 can (14 ounces/400 ml) coconut milk

1 cup (235 ml) water or chicken broth

1 can (4 ounces/113 g) mushroom stems and pieces, drained

2 to 3 chicken breasts, cut into bite-size pieces

1 jar (4 ounces/113 g) chopped pimiento

IN A LARGE SKILLET, heat the coconut oil over medium heat. Add the onion and bell pepper and sauté for about 6 minutes, until tender. Stir in the flour. Add the salt, pepper, coconut milk, water, mushrooms, chicken, and pimiento. Bring to a boil, then reduce the heat to medium-low and simmer, stirring frequently, for 10 minutes. Serve over hot biscuits, toast, mashed potatoes, rice, or noodles.   **SERVES 2 TO 3**

MUSHROOM À LA KING

Make the Chicken à La King (page 108) following the directions, but delete the chicken and canned mushrooms and use 8 ounces (70 g) of sliced fresh mushrooms. Cook the fresh mushrooms with the onion and bell pepper.

SAUSAGE À LA KING

Make Chicken à La King (page 108) according to the directions, but delete the chicken and add ½ pound (226 g) of sausage and 1 teaspoon of ground sage. Cook the sausage with the onion and bell pepper.

Creamy Chicken and Biscuits ⚙

2 tablespoons (30 ml) coconut oil

½ medium onion, finely chopped

1 rib celery, finely chopped

⅓ cup (42 g) flour

2 to 3 chicken breasts, cut into bite-size pieces

1 cup (235 g) water or chicken broth

1 can (14 ounces/400 ml) coconut milk

½ cup (75 g) peas

1 teaspoon salt

¼ teaspoon freshly ground black pepper

1 teaspoon ground sage

1 tablespoon (14 g) unsalted butter (optional)

Coconut Milk Biscuits (page 157)

IN A LARGE SKILLET, heat the coconut oil over medium heat. Add the onion and celery and sauté for about 6 minutes, until tender. Stir in the flour. Add the chicken, water, coconut milk, peas, salt, pepper, sage, and butter. Bring to a boil, then reduce the heat to low and simmer, stirring frequently, for 10 minutes. Serve over hot biscuits, toast, mashed potatoes, rice, or noodles. SERVES 2 TO 3

CREAMY TUNA AND BISCUITS
Make the Creamy Chicken and Biscuits (above) as directed, but omit the chicken and add 2 cans (6 ounces/170 g each) of tuna and 1 teaspoon of fish sauce. Fish sauce is salty, so you will need to reduce the amount of salt added. Fish sauce is available in the Asian section of the grocery store.
SERVES 2 TO 3

Ham and Potato Casserole

2 cans (14 ounces/400 ml each) coconut milk
½ cup (120 ml) water
½ cup (62 g) flour
1½ teaspoons salt
¾ teaspoon freshly ground black pepper
2 tablespoons (¼ stick/30 ml) unsalted butter or extra-virgin olive oil
5 to 6 potatoes, thinly sliced (about 6 cups/660 g)
1 medium onion, finely chopped
1 cup (150 g) finely chopped ham
2 cups (about 310 g) shredded cheese (cheddar works well)
Paprika

PREHEAT THE OVEN TO 375°F (190°C). In a large bowl, stir together the coconut milk, water, flour, salt, and pepper; set aside. Grease the bottom of a casserole dish with butter. Layer half of the potatoes on the bottom of the casserole dish, followed by half of the onion, half of the ham, half of the coconut milk mixture, and half of the cheese. Repeat the potato, onion, ham, coconut milk mixture, and cheese layering with the remaining half of the ingredients. Sprinkle the top with paprika. Cover and bake in the oven for 1 hour and 15 minutes. Uncover and bake 15 minutes more.   SERVES 4 TO 5

SPINACH, HAM, AND POTATO CASSEROLE
Make the Ham and Potato Casserole (above) as directed, but add 1 10-ounce (284-g) package of spinach. Thaw the spinach and squeeze out all of the liquid. Evenly layer all of the spinach on top of the first layer of potatoes.

Shepherd's Pie

1 pound (455 g) ground beef
½ cup (80 g) chopped onion
½ cup (75 g) chopped bell pepper
1 cup (8 ounces/70 g) chopped fresh mushrooms
1 cup (100 g) green beans
¼ cup (31 g) flour
1 can (14 ounces/400 ml) coconut milk
¼ cup (60 ml) water
1 teaspoon salt
⅛ teaspoon freshly ground black pepper
¼ cup (60 ml) tomato sauce
3 cups (about 630 g) hot Creamy Mashed Potatoes (page 136)
1 cup (about 155 g) shredded cheese
Paprika

PREHEAT THE OVEN TO 400°F (200°C). In a large skillet, brown the ground beef over medium heat. Add the onion, bell pepper, mushrooms, and green beans and cook for about 6 minutes, until tender. Stir in the flour. Add the coconut milk, water, salt, pepper, and tomato sauce. Heat, stirring frequently, for about 5 minutes, until the mixture thickens. Spoon the mixture into an ungreased 1½-quart (1½-liter) casserole dish, spread the potatoes over the surface, and roughen the surface with a fork. Sprinkle the top with cheese and paprika. Bake uncovered for 30 minutes. SERVES 3

Coconut Battered Shrimp

¾ cup (94 g) flour
¾ cup (175 ml) water
2 tablespoons (30 ml) tamari sauce
1 large egg
½ teaspoon onion powder
½ teaspoon salt, plus more to taste
⅛ teaspoon freshly ground black pepper, plus more to taste

Coconut oil for frying

½ pound (226 g) large shrimp, peeled and deveined, with tails left on

2 cups (170 g) flaked coconut

IN A MEDIUM BOWL, mix together the flour, water, tamari sauce, egg, onion powder, salt, and pepper. In a deep sauté pan, add the coconut oil to a depth of 1 inch and heat the oil to about 325°F (170°C) on a deep-fry thermometer. Pick up each shrimp by the tail, one at a time, and dip it in the batter, then coat evenly with the coconut. Deep-fry the shrimp in the hot oil for 3 to 4 minutes, until golden brown. Remove the shrimp and place on a paper towel–lined plate. Several shrimp can be cooked at the same time, depending on the size of the pan. Season to taste. This goes well with chutney, salsa, or chili sauce.   SERVES 2 TO 3

Jumbo Fried Coconut Shrimp

1 cup (125 g) flour

3 large eggs, beaten

¼ teaspoon cayenne pepper

1 teaspoon onion powder

1 teaspoon salt

3 cups (330 g) dried bread crumbs

1 cup (85 g) shredded coconut

24 large shrimp, peeled and deveined, with tails left on

Coconut oil for frying

IN A MEDIUM BOWL, place the flour. In a second bowl, combine the eggs, cayenne, onion powder, and salt. In a third bowl, mix together the bread crumbs and coconut. Holding the shrimp by the tail, dredge it in the flour, shaking off any excess, then dip it into the eggs, and finally roll it in the bread crumb mixture, coating each side. In a deep fryer or large saucepan, add the coconut oil to a depth of 1 inch and heat to 300°F (150°C) on a deep-fry thermometer. Fry the shrimp for about 3 minutes, until golden brown. Remove the shrimp and place on a paper towel–lined plate.

MAKES 24 FRIED SHRIMP

African Coconut Shrimp

¼ cup (60 ml) coconut oil

3 pounds (1.4 kg) shrimp, peeled, deveined, with tails removed

1 onion, finely chopped

4 cloves garlic, minced

3 sprigs of fresh parsley, finely chopped

2 large tomatoes, chopped

2 teaspoons crushed red pepper

2 teaspoons ground cumin

1 teaspoon salt

3 cups (710 ml) coconut milk

Hot cooked rice

IN A HEAVY SKILLET, heat the coconut oil over medium heat. Add the shrimp and cook for about 5 minutes, until pink. Remove the shrimp from the pan and set aside. In the same pan, add the onion, garlic, and parsley and sauté for 2 to 3 minutes, until the vegetables are slightly tender. Add the tomatoes, crushed red pepper, cumin, and salt. Cook, stirring constantly, for about 5 minutes, until the mixture thickens slightly. Reduce the heat to low and add the coconut milk and cooked shrimp. Cook and stir for about 4 minutes, until the shrimp is heated through. Serve over rice.   SERVES 6 TO 8

Shrimp and Asparagus in Coconut Sauce

3 tablespoons (45 ml) coconut oil

1 medium onion, chopped

1 bell pepper, chopped

1 pound (455 g) asparagus, chopped

2 tablespoons (15 g) flour

1 cup (235 ml) coconut milk

24 large shrimp

2 teaspoons fish sauce (see Note)

Salt and freshly ground black pepper to taste

IN A LARGE SKILLET, heat the coconut oil over medium heat. Add the onion and bell pepper and sauté for about 8 minutes, until the bell pepper is tender and the onion starts to brown. Add the asparagus along with the bell pepper and onion and cook, until the asparagus is tender and the onion starts to brown. In a small bowl, mix the flour with the coconut milk. Add the coconut milk mixture, the shrimp, and fish sauce to the vegetables and simmer for about 5 minutes, or until the shrimp is cooked and the sauce begins to thicken. Add salt and pepper to taste.   SERVES 3

Note
Tamari sauce can be substituted for fish sauce if you like.

ASIAN-STYLE CUISINE

Asian Spices

Coconuts grow throughout much of Asia, where they are extensively used in food preparation and cooking. Many of the classic or traditional foods associated with Thai and Indian cuisine involve coconut in one form or another. This chapter provides a variety of coconut-based meals inspired by traditional Asian dishes. Some of the meals are completely authentic while others are modified for ease of preparation using readily available ingredients.

Asian-style cuisine is characterized by its unique blend of exotic herbs and spices. People in non-Asian countries are often unfamiliar with many of the spices commonly used in Asian cooking, some of which can be hard to find outside their native countries. That isn't a problem with the recipes here. All of the spices and sauces used in this chapter can be found in your local grocery store, usually in the spice section. Some items, such as red curry paste and fish sauce, may be located in the Asian foods section. Such ingredients are also available at many health food stores and Asian markets. If you can't find them locally, they are available by mail.

Spices and sauces commonly used in Asian cooking that are included in this chapter are listed below.

Herbs and Spices

Cardamom	Cumin
Cayenne pepper	Curry powder
Chili powder	Garam masala
Cilantro	Garlic
Cinnamon	Ginger
Cloves	Lemongrass
Coriander	Mustard
Crushed red pepper	Turmeric

Sauces and Condiments

Chutney
Fish sauce
Green curry paste
Red chili paste
Red curry paste
Tahini (sesame seed butter)

Many Asian dishes are served with rice. Long-grain basmati rice is one of the most popular. I prefer short-grain brown rice. All of the dishes in this chapter may be made with any type of rice you prefer.

In Thailand, noodle dishes are popular. The most common noodles used in Thai cooking are rice noodles made from white rice flour. A variety of noodles made with other grains are also available, such as brown rice, whole wheat, corn, and spelt. You can use any of these noodles in the recipes that follow.

Fish sauce is the most popular seasoning in Thai cooking. It is made by extracting the juice from salted anchovies and is used much as you would use soy sauce. Because of its high salt content, additional salt is usually not needed. It has a pungent taste and aroma, which mellows when cooked. It adds a nice flavor to shrimp and other sea-food dishes. If fish sauce is not available, you can generally substitute soy sauce or tamari sauce.

Other common flavorings in Thai cooking are red or green curry paste and red chili paste. They can greatly enhance the flavor of foods. These pastes are hot, so be careful how much you use. If you put too much in a dish, you can temper the hotness by adding a little milk or yogurt.

Some Thai dishes are often called curries, but Indian food is characterized by its many flavorful and aromatic curries. Curries may contain any number or combination of seasonings including garam masala or curry powder. "Curry" is a term that has been applied to Asian, and particularly Indian, foods to describe any main dish or stew. Many curries contain no curry powder at all, yet they are still called curries. Curry powder isn't made from any single herb but is actually a blend of several different Indian spices such as coriander, turmeric, chili, cumin, and fenugreek. It is the turmeric that gives curry powder its distinctive mustard yellow color. Garam masala, like curry powder, is made from a blend of different spices including coriander, black pepper, cumin, cardamom, and cinnamon. Curries may or may not contain curry powder or garam masala.

Thai Chicken

> 1 3- to 4-inch (7- to 10-cm) hot red finger pepper (or other hot pepper)
> 2 tablespoons (30 ml) coconut oil
> 1 large clove garlic, minced
> 1½-inch (4-cm) piece ginger root, peeled and minced
> 1 medium onion, sliced
> 1 red bell pepper, seeded and sliced
> 1 green bell pepper, seeded and sliced
> 1 tablespoon (14 g) minced fresh lemongrass
> 1½ pounds (680 g) boneless, skinless chicken breast
> 1 tablespoon (15 ml) fish sauce
> ½ cup (120 ml) coconut milk
> ½ teaspoon red curry paste
> Salt to taste

REMOVE AND DISCARD the seeds from the hot red pepper and mince the hot pepper. In a large skillet, heat the coconut oil over medium heat. Add the garlic, ginger, and minced hot red pepper. Sauté for 2 minutes. Add the onion and cook for another 2 minutes. Add the bell peppers and lemongrass; cook for 2 minutes. Cut the chicken breasts in half and slice the halves into ½-inch (1.25-cm) slices; add to the skillet along with the fish sauce. Cook over medium-low heat, stirring frequently, for about 10 minutes, until the chicken becomes white and firm. Stir in the coconut milk and curry paste, add salt to taste, and cook for 2 to 3 minutes, until heated through.   SERVES 4

Indian-Style Lamb Stew

This thick stew can be served on a plate rather than in a bowl.

> 2 tablespoons (30 ml) coconut oil
> 1 small onion, chopped
> 6 cloves garlic, chopped
> 2 medium carrots, sliced
> 1 bell pepper, seeded and chopped
> 3 tablespoons (23 g) flour
> 2 cups (475 ml) water
> 1 can (14 ounces/400 ml) coconut milk
> 1½ pounds (680 g) lamb, cut into bite-size pieces
> 3 to 4 medium potatoes, chopped
> ¼ teaspoon ground cinnamon
> 1 teaspoon ground cardamom
> ¼ teaspoon ground cloves
> ½ teaspoon ground turmeric
> 1 teaspoon ground coriander
> ¼ teaspoon cayenne pepper
> 2 teaspoons salt

IN A LARGE SKILLET, heat the coconut oil over medium heat. Add the onion, garlic, carrots, and bell pepper and sauté for about 6 minutes, until the vegetables are tender. In a small bowl, mix the flour with the water; add the flour-water mixture, coconut milk, lamb, potatoes, cinnamon, cardamom, cloves, turmeric, coriander, cayenne, and salt to the vegetables and combine. Bring to a boil, then reduce the heat to low and simmer, stirring occasionally, for about 20 minutes, until the potatoes are tender.   SERVES 4

VARIATION
Instead of lamb, you can make this dish using chicken, pork, or shrimp.

Chicken in Curry Sauce

¼ cup (60 g) coconut oil

2 medium onions, thinly sliced

2 tablespoons (15 g) flour

1 teaspoon peeled, minced fresh ginger, or ½ teaspoon ground
     ginger

1 teaspoon minced garlic

3 pounds (1.4 kg) raw chicken, cut into small serving-size pieces

1 tablespoon (6 g) curry powder

½ teaspoon ground cumin

½ teaspoon ground coriander

1 teaspoon salt

½ teaspoon freshly ground black pepper

1 can (14 ounces/400 ml) coconut milk

¼ cup (60 g) chutney

½ cup (75 g) raisins

½ cup (68 g) roasted cashews

3 scallions (white and green parts), thinly sliced

Hot cooked rice

IN A LARGE frying pan with a tight-fitting lid, heat the coconut oil over medium heat. Add the onions and cook, uncovered, for about 4 minutes, until tender. Add the flour, ginger, and garlic and continue cooking, stirring occasionally, for about 4 minutes more, until the garlic is softened. Add the chicken pieces and cook for about 8 minutes, until evenly browned, turning once or twice. In a medium bowl, combine the curry powder, cumin, coriander, salt, pepper, coconut milk, and chutney and stir well. Scrape the mixture into the frying pan and turn the chicken and onion to combine well. Reduce the heat to low, cover, and simmer for about 45 minutes, turning the chicken once or twice, until it is tender and cooked through. Stir in the raisins and cashews, transfer the mixture to a serving dish, and sprinkle with the scallions. Serve with a side dish of rice.　SERVES 6

Chicken and Vegetables in Cream Sauce

This is a slightly modified version of a popular Indian recipe. A vegetarian version can be made by simply omitting the chicken. Green chili peppers give this dish a bit of a kick, which adds to the flavor. You can decrease the hotness of the dish by adjusting the number and type of peppers you use.

⅔ cup (153 g) plain yogurt

¼ cup (61 g) tomato sauce

2 tablespoons (30 ml) freshly squeezed lemon juice

1 teaspoon ground ginger

1 teaspoon chili powder

1 teaspoon ground coriander

1 teaspoon ground cumin

1 teaspoon dry mustard

1 teaspoon salt

2 tablespoons (30 g) peanut butter or tahini

1⅓ cups (315 ml) water

⅓ cup (80 ml) coconut oil

½ cup (80 g) chopped onion

4 cloves garlic, diced

1 to 4 hot chili peppers (depending how hot you want it)

8 to 10 cauliflower florets

1 carrot, sliced

4 small potatoes, cubed (about 2 cups/220 g)

4 boneless, skinless chicken breasts, cut into bite-size pieces

3 tablespoons (23 g) flour

1 cup (235 ml) coconut milk

2 tablespoons (2 g) chopped fresh cilantro

½ cup (115 g) cottage cheese

IN A LARGE BOWL, mix together the yogurt, tomato sauce, lemon juice, ginger, chili powder, coriander, cumin, mustard, salt, peanut butter, and

⅓ cup (80 ml) of the water. Set aside. In a large skillet with a tight-fitting lid, heat the coconut oil over medium heat. Add the onion and cook for about 4 minutes, until slightly tender. Add the garlic, chili peppers, cauliflower, carrot, and potatoes. Cover and cook, stirring occasionally, for about 10 minutes, until the potatoes are tender. Add the chicken, cover, and cook for 5 minutes more. Remove the cooked vegetables and chicken from the pan with a slotted spoon and set aside. Stir the flour into the remaining oil in the skillet and cook for about 4 minutes, until slightly browned. Pour in the yogurt and spice mixture, the coconut milk, and the remaining 1 cup (235 ml) of water. Cook, stirring constantly, for about 5 minutes, until the sauce comes to a boil and begins to thicken. Return the cooked vegetables and chicken to the pan, stirring gently to blend into the sauce. Stir in the cilantro and cottage cheese. Cook for about 2 minutes, until heated through.   SERVES 4

Potatoes and Green Beans in Coconut Sauce

In India this dish is called aloo phalli. Like many Indian curries, this recipe does not contain curry. "Curry" is a term used in the West to describe any type of Indian stew or main dish. One of the primary flavorings used in this recipe is garam masala. Garam masala is a combination of spices popularly used in Indian cooking. Like many Indian dishes, this one can be made with or without meat. This recipe includes chicken, but you can leave it out if you want. It makes a delightful vegetarian dish.

> 1 cup (230 g) plain yogurt
> ½ cup (120 ml) coconut milk
> 1½ teaspoons garam masala
> 1 teaspoon chili powder
> 1 teaspoon ground ginger
> ¼ teaspoon ground turmeric
> ¼ teaspoon ground cumin
> ¼ teaspoon ground cardamom
> 2 teaspoons salt
> ⅓ cup (80 ml) coconut oil
> 1 medium onion, chopped

4 cloves garlic, diced

3 to 4 medium potatoes, chopped

½ cup (50 g) sliced green beans

½ cauliflower, cut into florets

½ bell pepper, seeded and chopped

4 chicken breasts, cut into bite-size pieces

¾ cup (102 g) cashews

2 tablespoons (15 g) flour

1 tablespoon (1 g) chopped fresh cilantro

IN A 1-QUART BOWL, mix together the yogurt, coconut milk, garam masala, chili powder, ginger, turmeric, cumin, cardamom, and salt. Set aside. In a large skillet, heat the coconut oil over medium heat. Add the onion and sauté for about 4 minutes, until tender. Add the garlic, potatoes, green beans, cauliflower, and bell pepper. Cook, stirring occasionally, for about 10 minutes. Add the chicken, cashews, and flour. Cover and cook for 6 minutes. Stir in the yogurt mixture. Continue to cook, stirring occasionally, for about 1 to 2 minutes, until the mixture is hot. Stir in the cilantro and remove from the heat.

Like many curries, this dish goes well served with a side dish of fresh fruit. SERVES 4

Shrimp and Cauliflower in Coconut Sauce

⅓ cup (80 ml) coconut oil

1 medium onion, chopped

½ cup (55 g) slivered almonds

1 teaspoon ground coriander

2 teaspoons ground ginger

2 teaspoons curry powder

1 teaspoon salt

2 tablespoons (15 g) flour

4 cloves garlic, minced

1 to 3 chili peppers, seeded and chopped

½ cauliflower, cut into small florets

1 bell pepper, seeded and chopped

3 cups (680 g) shrimp

1 can (14 ounces/400 ml) coconut milk

2 tablespoons (2 g) chopped fresh cilantro

IN A LARGE SKILLET, heat the coconut oil over medium heat. Add the onion and sauté for about 5 minutes, until tender. Add the almonds and cook for 4 to 5 minutes, until slightly browned. Add the coriander, ginger, curry powder, salt, and flour and cook, stirring occasionally, for 4 minutes. Stir in the garlic, chili pepper, cauliflower, and bell pepper. Cover and cook for about 8 minutes, until the vegetables are tender. Add the shrimp, coconut milk, and cilantro. Stir constantly for about 6 minutes, until the sauce thickens and the shrimp is cooked.   SERVES 2 TO 3

Potato and Pea Korma

This is a delicious meatless dish from India. If desired, you could add chicken for a nonvegetarian version (see Note).

½ cup (115 g) plain yogurt

1 cup (235 ml) coconut milk

1 tablespoon (15 ml) freshly squeezed lemon juice

½ cup (122 g) tomato sauce

1 teaspoon salt

1 teaspoon garam masala

1 teaspoon ground ginger

1½ teaspoons ground coriander

1 teaspoon chili powder

½ teaspoon ground cardamom

⅛ teaspoon freshly ground black pepper

½ teaspoon ground cinnamon

⅓ cup (80 ml) coconut oil

2 tablespoons (18 g) sesame seeds

1 large onion, chopped

4 cloves garlic, chopped

2 to 3 potatoes, cubed

½ cup (50 g) sliced green beans

½ cup (75 g) peas

2 tomatoes

2 tablespoons (2 g) chopped fresh cilantro

IN A 1-QUART BOWL, mix together the yogurt, coconut milk, lemon juice, tomato sauce, salt, garam masala, ginger, coriander, chili powder, cardamom, pepper, and cinnamon and set aside. In a large skillet, heat the coconut oil over medium heat. Add the sesame seeds and onion and sauté for about 5 minutes, until the onion is tender. Add the garlic, potatoes, green beans, and peas. Cook, stirring occasionally, for about 10 minutes, until the green vegetables are tender. Stir in the yogurt mixture and simmer for about 8 minutes, until the potatoes are tender but not mushy. Cut each tomato into 10 to 12 wedges. Add the tomato wedges and cilantro to the skillet and cook for 1 minute. Remove the skillet from the heat and serve. This dish goes well served with a side dish of fried okra (see under Fried Vegetables, page 144).   SERVES 2 TO 3

Note

For the nonvegetarian version, add 4 chicken breasts cut into bite-size pieces. Put the chicken in the skillet along with the yogurt and cook as directed.

Pineapple Shrimp in Coconut Milk

2 tablespoons (30 ml) coconut oil

2 cups (200 g) sliced cauliflower

1 medium carrot, sliced

½ cup (80 g) chopped onion

2 tablespoons (15 g) flour

1 can (14 ounces/400 ml) coconut milk

1 teaspoon salt

⅛ teaspoon freshly ground black pepper

1 tablespoon (5.5 g) ground ginger

½ pound (226 g) medium-size shrimp, shelled

1½ cups (250 g) fresh pineapple chunks

Hot cooked rice

IN A LARGE SAUCEPAN, heat the coconut oil over medium heat. Add the cauliflower, carrot, and onion and sauté for about 6 minutes, until tender.

Add the flour and cook for 1 minute. Add the coconut milk, salt, pepper, and ginger. Reduce the heat to low and simmer, covered, for 10 minutes. Raise the heat to high and add the shrimp. Cook for about 1 minute, or until the shrimp turn pink. Add the pineapple and cook 1 minute more. Remove from the heat. Serve over hot cooked rice.   SERVES 2

Peanut Chicken

> 1 tablespoon (15 ml) coconut oil
> 1½ pounds (680 g) chicken, cut into 1-inch (2.5-cm) pieces
> 1 onion, chopped
> 1 red bell pepper, chopped
> 1 medium zucchini, sliced
> 1 tablespoon (8 g) flour
> 1 can (14 ounces/400 ml) coconut milk
> Freshly squeezed juice of 1 lemon
> ½ cup (130 g) salsa
> 1 tablespoon (15 g) red chili paste
> 1 teaspoon salt
> ¾ cup (195 g) chunky peanut butter
> Hot cooked rice

IN A LARGE SKILLET, heat the coconut oil over medium heat. Add the chicken, onion, bell pepper, and zucchini; cook for about 6 minutes, until the vegetables are tender. Stir in the flour. Add the coconut milk, lemon juice, salsa, chili paste, salt, and peanut butter. Reduce the heat to low and simmer for 10 minutes. Serve over hot cooked rice.   SERVES 4 TO 5

Apple and Sweet Potato Curry

This recipe can serve as a vegetarian main course or as a great side dish.

> 3 tablespoons (45 ml) coconut oil
> 1 medium sweet potato or yam, cut into bite-size pieces
> 1 medium onion, chopped
> 1 teaspoon ground mustard

1½ teaspoons ground cumin

1 teaspoon ground coriander

½ teaspoon ground turmeric

1 teaspoon salt

2 cloves garlic, minced

2 tart apples, peeled, cored, and sliced

½ cup (75 g) raisins

1 can (14 ounces/400 ml) coconut milk

¼ cup (21 g) flaked or shredded coconut

IN A LARGE SKILLET, heat the coconut oil over medium heat. Add the sweet potato and onion and sauté for about 8 minutes, until the onion is tender. Add the mustard, cumin, coriander, turmeric, salt, and garlic and cook for 2 minutes. Stir in the apples, raisins, coconut milk, and coconut. Cover and simmer for about 12 minutes, until the sweet potato is tender.

SERVES 2

Chicken in Red Curry Sauce

¼ cup (60 ml) coconut oil

4 to 6 chicken thighs, boned and halved

3 tablespoons (42 g) red curry paste

2 cups (475 ml) water

1 can (14 ounces/400 ml) coconut milk

1 sweet potato, cut into bite-size pieces

¼ cup (4 g) chopped fresh cilantro

IN A LARGE SKILLET, heat the coconut oil over medium heat. Add the chicken, cover, and cook the chicken for 5 minutes. Turn the chicken and cook for another 5 minutes. Add the red curry paste, water, coconut milk, and sweet potato. Reduce the heat to low, cover, and simmer for about 15 minutes, or until the sweet potato is tender and the sauce is thickened. Uncover, add the cilantro, and cook for 2 minutes more.   SERVES 2 TO 3

Thai Coconut Shrimp and Noodles ⚙

8 ounces (38 g) noodles

3 tablespoons (45 ml) coconut oil

1 cup (160 g) chopped onion

2 tablespoons (30 g) seeded and chopped green chili peppers

4 cloves garlic, minced

1 tablespoon (8 g) flour

1 can (14 ounces/400 ml) coconut milk

2 tablespoons (30 ml) fish sauce

½ pound (226 g) shrimp, peeled and deveined

2 tablespoons (2 g) finely chopped fresh cilantro

PREPARE THE NOODLES according to the package directions; drain and set aside. (Traditionally rice noodles are most commonly used in Thai cooking, but you can use any type of noodle you like.) In a large skillet, heat the coconut oil over medium heat. Add the onion and sauté for about 6 minutes, until tender. Add the green chili, garlic, and flour and continue to cook, stirring frequently, for 3 minutes. Stir in the coconut milk and fish sauce and simmer uncovered, stirring occasionally, for about 8 minutes, until the sauce thickens. Add the shrimp and cilantro and continue to simmer until the shrimp is cooked, 3 to 4 minutes. Remove from the heat and fold in the noodles until well coated with sauce. Serve hot.   SERVES 2 TO 3

Red Thai Curry

1 pound (455 g) noodles

2 tablespoons (30 ml) coconut oil

1 onion, chopped

4 cloves garlic, minced

2 carrots, sliced

1 red bell pepper, seeded and diced

1 tablespoon (6 g) ground ginger

1 tablespoon (8 g) flour

1 can (14 ounces/400 ml) coconut milk

1 tablespoon (14 g) red curry paste (see Note)

2 tablespoons (30 ml) fish sauce or soy sauce

1 pound (455 g) shrimp, peeled and deveined

¼ cup (4 g) finely chopped fresh cilantro, for garnish

PREPARE THE NOODLES according to the package directions; drain and set aside. In a large skillet, heat the coconut oil over medium heat. Add the onion and garlic and sauté for about 5 minutes, until tender. Add the carrots, bell pepper, and ginger and sauté for about 7 minutes, until the vegetables are soft. In a small bowl, mix the flour with the coconut milk. Add the coconut milk mixture, curry paste, and fish sauce to the skillet and cook until the curry paste is well blended. Add the shrimp, reduce the heat to low, and simmer for 3 to 4 minutes, until the shrimp is pink. Remove the skillet from the heat and fold in the noodles until they are well coated with sauce. Garnish with the cilantro.   SERVES 4

Note
Red curry paste is hot. You may adjust the spiciness of this dish by increasing or reducing the amount of curry paste used. If you find that you have used too much, you can reduce the hotness by adding a little milk or yogurt.

Lamb and Squash Curry

¼ cup (60 ml) coconut oil

1 onion, chopped

4 cloves garlic, chopped

2 potatoes, cubed

1 carrot, sliced

1 fresh green chili, seeded and chopped

1 pound (455 g) lamb, cubed (see Note)

1 large zucchini or yellow squash, sliced

2 tablespoons (12 g) ground coriander

1 tablespoon (7 g) chili powder

1 teaspoon ground cumin

1 teaspoon ground ginger

1 teaspoon ground turmeric

2 teaspoons curry powder

1 tablespoon ground mustard

2 teaspoons salt

1 cup (235 ml) water

3 tablespoons (23 g) flour

1 can (14 ounces/400 ml) coconut milk

¼ cup (60 ml) apple cider vinegar

IN A LARGE SKILLET, heat the coconut oil over medium heat. Add the onion and garlic and sauté for about 5 minutes, until tender. Add the potatoes, carrot, and green chili. Cover and cook, stirring occasionally, for 5 to 7 minutes, until the vegetables are partially tender. Add the lamb, zucchini, coriander, chili powder, cumin, ginger, turmeric, curry powder, ground mustard, salt, and water and simmer for about 12 minutes, until the potatoes are tender. In a small bowl, mix the flour with the coconut milk; add the mixture to the skillet along with the vinegar. Cook for about 5 minutes, until the mixture thickens. SERVES 3 TO 4

Note

Pork may be substituted for the lamb if you wish.

Gingered Sweet Potatoes in Coconut Sauce ⚙

This recipe makes a good meatless main course or side dish.

3 tablespoons (45 ml) coconut oil

1 onion, diced

1 tablespoon (5.5 g) ground ginger

1 tablespoon (6 g) curry powder

1 can (14 ounces/400 ml) coconut milk

1 large sweet potato, cut into bite-size pieces

1 cup (165 g) chopped fresh pineapple

1 tablespoon (15 ml) tamari sauce

1 teaspoon salt

IN A LARGE SAUCEPAN, heat the coconut oil over medium heat. Add the onion and sauté for about 6 minutes, until tender. Mix in the ginger and curry powder and cook for another 1 to 2 minutes, until fragrant. Add the coconut milk, sweet potatoes, pineapple, tamari sauce, and salt. Reduce the heat to low, cover, and simmer for 25 to 30 minutes, until the sweet potatoes are soft but still firm enough to keep their shape.   SERVES 2

Potato and Spinach Curry

3 tablespoons (45 ml) coconut oil

4 red potatoes, diced

1 onion, chopped

4 cloves garlic, minced

1 can (14 ounces/400 ml) coconut milk

1 tablespoon (5.5 g) ground ginger

1 teaspoon ground cumin

2 teaspoons (14 g) ground turmeric

2 teaspoons salt

1 10-ounce (284 g) package frozen chopped spinach (see Note)

1 large tomato, diced

¼ cup (4 g) minced fresh cilantro

IN A LARGE SKILLET, heat the coconut oil over medium heat. Add the potatoes, onion, and garlic. Cover and cook for 10 minutes. Reduce the heat to low. Add the coconut milk, ginger, cumin, turmeric, and salt. Simmer for about 10 minutes, until the potatoes are tender but still hold their shape. Add the spinach and tomato and cook for 2 minutes more. Serve garnished with the cilantro.   SERVES 2

Note

One half-pound (226 g) of fresh spinach can be substituted for the frozen spinach if desired.

Peanut Butter Pork

1 cup (235 ml) coconut milk

½ cup (130 g) chunky peanut butter

1 tablespoon (15 g) red chili paste

1 tablespoon (15 ml) freshly squeezed lemon juice

1 teaspoon ground ginger

1 teaspoon salt

2 tablespoons (30 ml) coconut oil

1 pound (455 g) pork, cut into bite-size pieces

1 medium onion, chopped

2 cloves garlic, diced

½ red bell pepper, seeded and diced

Noodles

IN A LARGE BOWL, combine the coconut milk, peanut butter, red chili paste, lemon juice, ginger, and salt. Mix together and set aside. In a large skillet, heat the coconut oil over medium heat. Add the pork and sauté for about 4 minutes, until it is barely cooked through. Add the onion, garlic, and bell pepper and continue to cook for about 8 minutes, until the vegetables are tender and the meat is thoroughly cooked. Stir in the coconut milk mixture, reduce the heat to low, and simmer for 4 or 5 minutes, until the mixture is hot. Serve over a bed of hot noodles.   SERVES 2 TO 3

Coconut-Seafood Stew ✿

1½ cups (355 ml) chicken broth or water

½ onion, diced

1 potato, chopped

1 8-ounce (226-g) fresh fish fillet, with skin on (see Note)

1 10-ounce (284-g) package frozen spinach

¼ teaspoon ground ginger

½ teaspoon ground coriander

1½ teaspoons fish sauce

½ teaspoon green curry paste

1 can (14 ounces/400 ml) coconut milk

¼ teaspoon salt

8 ounces (226 g) shrimp

Freshly squeezed juice of half a lime

IN A LARGE SAUCEPAN, heat the chicken broth over medium heat. Add the onion, potato, and fish fillet and simmer for about 10 minutes, until the fish is cooked through. Remove the fish fillet. Add the spinach, ginger, coriander, fish sauce, green curry paste, coconut milk, and salt and simmer for about 10 minutes, or until the potato is tender. Remove the skin from the fish fillet and cut or break the fish into ½-inch pieces. Add the fish and shrimp to the saucepan and cook for about 3 minutes more, until the shrimp is cooked. Remove from the heat and add the lime juice. Serve in bowls.   SERVES 4

Note
You can use any type of white fish.

Coconut-Chicken Soup ❀

4 cups (950 ml) water
½ medium onion, chopped
3 cloves garlic, chopped
3 chicken breasts, cut into bite-size pieces
1 large tomato, chopped
1½ tablespoons (25 ml) fish sauce
1 teaspoon curry powder
1 teaspoon ground ginger
1 teaspoon salt
1 can (14 ounces/400 ml) coconut milk
1 pound (455 g) chopped fresh spinach (see Note)
¼ cup (4 g) chopped fresh cilantro

IN A LARGE SAUCEPAN, bring the water to a boil over medium heat. Add the onion, garlic, chicken, tomato, fish sauce, curry powder, ginger, and salt. Reduce the heat to medium-low, cover, and simmer for 15 minutes. Add the coconut milk and spinach and cook for 5 minutes more. Remove from the heat and add the cilantro.   SERVES 2 TO 3

Note
One 10-ounce (284 g) package of frozen chopped spinach can be substituted for fresh spinach if desired.

Chicken and Sweet Potato Stew with Coconut Dumplings

4 cups (950 ml) chicken broth

3 chicken breasts, cut into bite-size pieces

½ onion, chopped

6 cloves garlic, chopped

1 medium sweet potato, chopped (3 cups)

1 cup (150 g) peas

1½ teaspoons salt

2 teaspoons curry powder

½ teaspoon garam masala

1 teaspoon ground cardamom

⅛ teaspoon freshly ground black pepper

1 tablespoon (8 g) flour

1 can (14 ounces/400 ml) coconut milk

Coconut Dumplings (recipe below)

IN A LARGE SAUCEPAN, bring the broth to a boil over medium heat. Add the chicken, onion, garlic, sweet potato, peas, salt, curry powder, garam masala, cardamom, and pepper. Reduce the heat to low and simmer for about 20 minutes, until the sweet potato is barely tender. In a small bowl, mix the flour with the coconut milk then stir the mixture into the stew. Drop the Coconut Dumplings into the stew, cover, and simmer for 15 minutes. Serve in bowls.   SERVES 3 TO 4

Coconut Dumplings

1 cup (125 g) flour, plus more for coating the dumplings

½ cup (42 g) grated coconut

½ teaspoon onion powder

¼ cup (4 g) diced fresh cilantro

½ teaspoon salt

1½ teaspoons baking powder

½ cup (120 ml) coconut milk

1 large egg

IN A LARGE BOWL, mix together the flour, coconut, onion powder, cilantro, salt, and baking powder. In a separate bowl, mix together the coconut milk and egg. Combine the wet ingredients and the dry ingredients. Form the dough into 1-inch (2.5-cm) balls. Coat each one with flour and drop into the stew.   MAKES 12 DUMPLINGS

Burmese Peanut Chicken

2 teaspoons (30 ml) coconut oil

1 chicken (3 to 4 pounds/1.4 to 1.8 kg), cut into serving-size pieces

1 medium yellow onion, chopped

1 carrot, sliced

1 rib celery, sliced

3 cloves garlic, minced

¼ teaspoon ground cinnamon

½ teaspoon ground ginger

Dash of cayenne pepper

⅛ teaspoon ground cloves

1 teaspoon salt

3 tablespoons (45 ml) soy sauce

½ cup (130 g) chunky peanut butter

1 can (14 ounces/400 ml) coconut milk

Hot cooked rice

IN A HEAVY SKILLET, heat the coconut oil over medium heat. Add the chicken and brown well on all sides. Add the onion, carrot, celery, and garlic and cook for 4 to 5 minutes, until slightly tender. Mix in the cinnamon, ginger, cayenne, cloves, salt, soy sauce, peanut butter, and coconut milk. Cover, reduce the heat to medium-low, and simmer for 20 minutes, or until the chicken is done. Serve over hot cooked rice.   SERVES 4

SIDE DISHES

Creamy Scalloped Potatoes

Coconut oil or butter, for greasing the casserole dish

1 can (14 ounces/400 ml) coconut milk

½ cup (120 ml) water

¼ cup (31 g) flour

2 teaspoons salt

¼ teaspoon freshly ground black pepper

4 to 6 potatoes, thinly sliced

1 medium onion, finely chopped

1 red or green bell pepper, seeded and chopped

2 cups (about 310 g) grated cheese

Paprika

PREHEAT THE OVEN TO 350°F (180°C). Grease the bottom of a casserole dish with coconut oil. In a medium bowl, stir together the coconut milk, water, flour, salt, and pepper; set aside. Layer half of the potatoes on the bottom of the casserole, followed by half of the onion, half of the bell pepper, half of the cheese, and half of the coconut milk mixture. Repeat the potato, onion, bell pepper, cheese, and coconut milk mixture, layering with the remaining half of the ingredients. Sprinkle the top with paprika. Bake for about 1 hour and 15 minutes, or until the potatoes are tender. SERVES 6

Creamy Mashed Potatoes

> 6 medium potatoes (2 pounds/1 kg)
> ⅓ to ½ cup (80 to 120 ml) coconut milk
> ½ teaspoon salt, plus more to taste
> Dash of freshly ground black pepper, plus more to taste

CHOP THE POTATOES into ½-inch (1.25-cm) pieces and put them into a large suacepan. Add just enough water to cover the potatoes. Cover, bring to a boil over medium heat, and cook for about 25 to 30 minutes, until tender. Drain. Mash the potatoes, adding coconut milk a little at a time, until smooth and fluffy. (The amount of coconut milk needed depends on the variety of potato.) Add salt and pepper to taste.   SERVES 6

GARLIC MASHED POTATOES
Cook the potatoes as directed in Creamy Mashed Potatoes (above). After draining the water, add 6 to 10 crushed cloves of garlic, ½ teaspoon of onion powder, salt, and pepper. Mix the ingredients, cover, and let stand for 5 minutes. Mash with enough coconut milk for a good consistency. Before serving, sprinkle with paprika or chives if desired.

LEMON MASHED POTATOES
Make the Creamy Mashed Potatoes (above) as directed. Stir in 1 tablespoon (15 ml) of freshly squeezed lemon juice when adding the salt and pepper.

MEXICAN MASHED POTATOES
Make the Creamy Mashed Potatoes (above) as directed. Stir ½ cup (130 g) of salsa into the mashed potatoes.

CHEESY MASHED POTATOES
Make the Creamy Mashed Potatoes (above) as directed. Stir 1 cup (235 ml) of Thick Cheddar Cheese Sauce (page 63) into the mashed potatoes. Sprinkle the top with paprika.

BACON AND CHEESE POTATOES

Make the Creamy Mashed Potatoes (page 136) as directed. Serve with Creamy Cheese Sauce (page 63) poured over the potatoes like gravy and topped with crumbled bacon.

FRIED MASHED POTATOES

This is a good way to use leftover mashed potatoes. Combine 1 cup (210 g) of cold mashed potatoes, 1 slightly beaten egg, ¼ cup (40 g) of diced onion, ½ teaspoon of salt, and ¼ teaspoon of pepper. Mix well. Shape into 6 patties. In a large skillet, heat 2 tablespoons (30 ml) of coconut oil over medium-high heat. Add the patties and cook, browning both sides.   MAKES 4 TO 6 PATTIES

Super Baked Potato

PREHEAT THE OVEN to 400°F (200°C). Scrub a potato well and pierce it several times with a fork or sharp knife to allow steam to escape. Bake it directly on the oven racks for 1 hour. Cut the potato lengthwise in half. Top with Thick Cheddar Cheese Sauce (page 63) or Tex-Mex Cheddar Cheese Sauce (page 63), salt and pepper, diced scallions (white and green parts), and crumbled bacon. You might also enjoy adding a little dill, basil, parsley, or marjoram.   SERVES 1

Twice-Baked Potato ✿

PREHEAT THE OVEN to 400°F (200°C). Prepare and bake the potato as described in Super Baked Potato (above). Remove the potato from the oven and let it cool. Raise the oven temperature to 450°F (230°C). As soon as the potato is cool enough to handle, cut the potato in half lengthwise. Scoop out the center without damaging the skin, leaving a thin shell. Mash the scooped-out portion of the potato along with ½ cup (120 ml) of Thick Cheddar Cheese Sauce (page 63), 1 tablespoon (15 ml) of freshly squeezed lemon juice, ½ teaspoon of salt, and a dash of pepper for each potato prepared. Blend all of the ingredients together until the mixture becomes creamy. Mound the mixture into each half of the potato shell. Return the potato to the oven and cook for about 15 minutes, or until the top of the potato filling begins to brown. Remove from the oven and serve. Top with chopped chives or scallions. SERVES 1

VARIATION
Make as directed, but replace the Thick Cheddar Cheese Sauce with Shrimp Cheese Sauce (page 64).

Mashed Sweet Potato

1 cup (235 ml) coconut milk
1 tart apple, cored, peeled, and chopped
2 tablespoons (40 g) honey or maple syrup
1½ teaspoons ground cinnamon
¼ teaspoon ground nutmeg
½ teaspoon salt
1 large sweet potato, cooked until soft (see Note)
Toasted coconut or almonds, for garnish

IN A SMALL SAUCEPAN, combine the coconut milk, apple, honey, cinnamon, nutmeg, and salt. Simmer over low heat for about 5 minutes, until the apple is soft; do not boil. Remove and discard the skin of the sweet potato; mash the sweet potato thoroughly. Add the mashed sweet potato to the coconut milk mixture. Serve hot. Garnish with toasted coconut or almonds.
SERVES 2

Note
You may substitute 1 medium butternut squash for the sweet potato, if desired.

Creamed Corn

3 tablespoons (42 g) unsalted butter
½ medium onion, chopped
½ cup (75 g) diced green bell pepper
2 tablespoons (15 g) flour

1 can (14 ounces/400 ml) coconut milk

3 cups (498 g) whole kernel corn (fresh or canned)

1 teaspoon salt

¼ teaspoon freshly ground black pepper

IN A LARGE SAUCEPAN, melt the butter over medium heat. Add the onion and bell pepper and sauté for about 8 minutes, until the vegetables are tender. Stir in the flour and cook for 2 minutes. Add the coconut milk, corn, salt, and pepper. Bring to a boil, reduce the heat to medium-low, and simmer for 4 to 5 minutes, until the mixture thickens.   SERVES 4

Creamed Peas

2 tablespoons (¼ stick/28 g) unsalted butter

½ medium onion, chopped

2 tablespoons (15 g) flour

1 can (14 ounces/400 ml) coconut milk

2½ cups (375 g) peas

½ teaspoon salt

¼ teaspoon freshly ground black pepper

IN A MEDIUM SAUCEPAN, melt the butter over medium heat. Add the onion and sauté for 8 minutes, until tender. Stir in the flour and cook for 2 minutes. Add the coconut milk, peas, salt, and pepper. Bring to a boil, reduce the heat to medium-low, and simmer for 4 to 5 minutes, until the mixture thickens.   SERVES 3 TO 4

CURRIED PEAS

Make the Creamed Peas (above) as directed, and add 1 teaspoon of curry powder.   SERVES 3 TO 4

Creamed Vegetables with Fish Sauce

2 tablespoons (¼ stick/28 g) unsalted butter or coconut oil

½ medium onion, chopped

2 tablespoons (15 g) flour

1 can (14 ounces/400 ml) coconut milk

3 cups (about 390 g) vegetables (see Note)

½ teaspoon fish sauce

Salt and freshly ground black pepper to taste

IN A LARGE SAUCEPAN, heat the butter over medium heat. Add the onion and sauté for about 6 minutes, until tender. Stir in the flour and cook for 2 minutes. Add the coconut milk, vegetables, fish sauce, salt, and pepper. Bring to a boil, reduce the heat to medium-low, and simmer for about 15 minutes, until the mixture thickens and the vegetables are tender.   SERVES 2 TO 3

Note

You can use any one of the following vegetables or any combination of them: asparagus, carrots, peas, green beans, broccoli, Brussels sprouts, cauliflower, lima beans, corn, and zucchini.

Spicy Creamed Spinach

1 tablespoon (15 ml) coconut oil

½ large onion, finely diced

½ teaspoon ground cumin

¼ teaspoon ground cardamom

¼ teaspoon ground turmeric

¼ teaspoon ground ginger

½ teaspoon salt

10 ounces (284 g) fresh spinach

½ cup (120 ml) coconut milk

IN A LARGE SKILLET, heat the coconut oil over medium heat. Add the onion and cook for about 6 minutes, until tender. Add the cumin, cardamom, turmeric, ginger, and salt and cook for about 1 minute, until the spices release their flavors. Add the spinach, cover, and cook for 1 to 2 minutes, until slightly wilted. Pour in the coconut milk and cook uncovered until the spinach is completely cooked, but do not overcook. Serve hot.   SERVES 2 TO 3

Cardamom Rice

> 1 cup (190 g) brown rice
> 1 cup (235 ml) water
> 1 can (14 ounces/400 ml) coconut milk
> ½ teaspoon ground cardamom
> ¼ teaspoon ground cinnamon
> ¼ teaspoon salt

IN A MEDIUM SAUCEPAN, combine the rice and the water and soak the rice for at least 4 hours. Add the coconut milk, cardamom, cinnamon, and salt. Bring to a boil over medium-high heat, reduce the heat to medium-low, cover, and simmer for about 45 minutes, or until the rice is tender and the liquid is absorbed. This goes well with fish, lamb, or chicken.   SERVES 2

Sesame Zucchini ☙

> ¼ cup (60 ml) coconut oil
> 2 tablespoons (18 g) sesame
>   seeds
> ½ cup (80 g) diced onion
> 2 cloves garlic, diced
>
> 2 medium zucchini, sliced
> ¼ teaspoon ground ginger
> ½ teaspoon salt
> 2 tablespoons (30 ml)
>   tamari sauce

IN A LARGE SKILLET, heat the coconut oil over medium heat. Add the sesame seeds and toast them in the coconut oil for about 3 minutes, until lightly browned. Add the onion and garlic and cook, stirring occasionally, for 3 to 4 minutes. Add the zucchini, cover, and cook until tender. Mix in the ginger and salt. Remove from the heat and add the tamari sauce. Include some of the drippings from the pan with each serving.   SERVES 2 TO 4

Vegetables with Cheese Sauce

Make the Creamy Cheese Sauce (page 63) and pour over steamed or sautéed vegetables. The sauce tastes great with asparagus, broccoli, cauliflower, zucchini, Brussels sprouts, potatoes, onions, peas, or bell peppers.

Macaroni and Cheese

 3 cups (420 g) cooked elbow macaroni
 1½ cups (355 ml) Creamy Cheese Sauce (page 63)
 1 tablespoon (3 g) finely chopped fresh chives, for garnish

COOK THE MACARONI according to the package directions. Drain the macaroni and mix in the Creamy Cheese Sauce. Garnish with fresh chives.
SERVES 2

BEEF MACARONI AND CHEESE
In a large skillet, cook ½ pound (226 g) of ground beef and ½ medium onion over medium heat for about 15 minutes, until the meat is browned and the onion is soft. Mix into the Macaroni and Cheese recipe (above). SERVES 2

Shrimp Macaroni and Cheese

Make the Macaroni and Cheese recipe (above) according to the directions, but substitute Shrimp Cheese Sauce (page 64) for the Creamy Cheese Sauce. SERVES 2

Cheese Cups ⚙

This delicious bread pudding is filled with cheese and bacon. It makes a great breakfast or side dish at dinner. The Fruit Cups described below are suitable for breakfast or as an after-dinner dessert.

 3 strips bacon
 1 large egg
 ½ cup (120 ml) coconut milk
 ½ cup (62 g) flour
 ¼ teaspoon salt
 ½ cup (120 ml) Creamy Cheese Sauce (page 63)
 Chives

PREHEAT THE OVEN TO 425°F (220°C). In a medium skillet, cook the bacon for about 8 minutes, until crisp; set it aside but reserve the drippings. In the bowl of a blender, mix the egg, coconut milk, flour, and salt at high speed for about 1 minute, until the mixture is bubbly. Coat the bottom of a 6-cup muffin pan generously with bacon drippings. Pour the egg mixture into the cups and bake for 18 minutes. Remove from the oven. Each pudding cup will have a slight depression in the center. Generously fill each depression with warm Creamy Cheese Sauce and top with crumbled bacon and chives. Serve hot.   MAKES 6 CHEESE CUPS

CRAB CUPS

Make the Cheese Cups (page 142) as directed, but replace the Creamy Cheese Sauce with Crab Cheese Sauce (page 63). Garnish with chives.

SHRIMP CUPS

Make the Cheese Cups (page 142) as directed, but replace the Creamy Cheese Sauce with the Shrimp Cheese Sauce (page 64).

FRUIT CUPS

Make the Cheese Cups (page 142) as directed, but omit the bacon, coat the muffin pan with coconut oil or butter, and replace the Creamy Cheese Sauce with a Fruit Sauce (page 60).

Onion Fritters ❁

>1 cup (235 ml) coconut milk
>¼ cup (60 ml) water
>1 large egg
>¾ cup (94 g) flour
>1 teaspoon onion powder
>½ teaspoon salt, plus more for sprinkling
>1 large Spanish or Bermuda onion, chopped into small pieces
>Coconut oil for deep-frying

IN A LARGE BOWL, mix together the coconut milk, water, egg, flour, onion powder, and salt until smooth. Stir the onion into the batter. In a deep fryer or large saucepan, add the coconut oil to a depth of 2 inches. Heat the oil to 325 to 350°F (170 to 180°C) on a deep-fry thermometer. Drop the batter by the spoonful into the hot oil. Fry a few spoonfuls at a time until golden brown. Drain on a paper towel–lined plate. Sprinkle with salt while still hot. Keep warm in a hot (200°F/90°C) oven until ready to serve.

MAKES 12 FRITTERS

FRIED VEGETABLES

Follow the directions for making Onion Fritters (page 143), but substitute other vegetables for the onion. Vegetables that fry well include okra, cauliflower, carrot, mushrooms, zucchini, and yams.

French Fries

PEEL AND CUT POTATOES lengthwise into thin strips. Fill a deep fryer or large saucepan half full with coconut oil and heat to 325 to 350°F (170 to 180°C) on a deep-fry thermometer. Fry the potato strips a few at a time for about 8 minutes, or until they are lightly golden and the insides are tender. Drain on a paper towel–lined plate. Sprinkle with salt while still hot. Keep warm in a hot (200°F/90°C) oven until ready to serve.

YIELD VARIES, DEPENDING ON HOW MANY POTATOES YOU USE

Cheese Nachos

GREAT-TASTING CHEESE Nachos can be made using Coconut Tortilla Corn Chips (recipe below) and Tex-Mex Cheddar Cheese Sauce (page 63). Just pour the cheese sauce over the corn chips and enjoy. These also taste good combined with ground beef and/or refried beans.

YIELD VARIES, DEPENDING ON HOW MANY TORTILLAS YOU USE

Coconut Tortilla Corn Chips

FILL A DEEP FRYER or large saucepan half full with coconut oil and heat to 325 to 350°F (170 to 180°C) on a deep-fry thermometer. Cut each corn tortilla into four equal pieces. Cook in the hot oil for about 2 minutes, until crisp. Place on a paper towel–lined plate to drain. Sprinkle the fried tortillas with a pinch of salt while still hot.

YIELD VARIES, DEPENDING ON HOW MANY TORTILLAS YOU USE

BREADS AND GRAINS

Coconut-Bran Muffins

Coconut oil, for greasing the muffin pan

1 cup (125 g) whole-wheat flour, plus more for dusting the muffin pan

1 cup (235 ml) water

1 tablespoon (15 ml) vanilla extract

⅓ cup (115 g) honey

1 large egg

¼ cup (25 g) wheat bran

¼ cup (21 g) grated coconut

2 teaspoons baking powder

¼ teaspoon salt

1 teaspoon ground cinnamon

½ teaspoon ground nutmeg

¼ cup (60 ml) coconut oil, melted

½ cup (about 67 g) almonds, pecans, or walnuts

PREHEAT THE OVEN TO 400°F (200°C). Coat a muffin pan with a thin layer of coconut oil and dust with flour. In a medium bowl, combine the water, vanilla, honey, egg, and bran and let sit for about 10 minutes. The bran will absorb some of the moisture as it sits, which will improve the texture of the final product. In another bowl, mix the flour, coconut, baking powder, salt, cinnamon, and nutmeg. Add the melted (not hot) coconut oil to the liquid ingredients. Then add the nuts and mix together. Combine the wet ingredients and the dry ingredients in one bowl and mix just until moist. Do not overmix or the muffins will not rise as well. Fill the muffin cups about half full. Bake for 15 minutes, or until a toothpick inserted in the center comes out clean.   MAKES 12 MUFFINS

Coconutty Muffins

Coconut oil for greasing the muffin pan
1 cup (125 g) whole-wheat flour, plus more for dusting the muffin pan
1 cup (235 ml) water
1 teaspoon vanilla extract
½ teaspoon almond extract
⅓ cup (115 g) honey
1 large egg
½ cup (42 g) grated coconut
2 teaspoons baking powder
¼ teaspoon salt
¼ cup (60 ml) coconut oil, melted
½ cup (about 55 g) almonds, pecans, or walnuts

PREHEAT THE OVEN TO 400°F (200°C). Coat a muffin pan with a thin layer of coconut oil and dust with flour. In a medium bowl, combine the water, vanilla, almond extract, honey, and egg and set aside. In another bowl, mix together the flour, coconut, baking powder, and salt. Add the melted (not hot) coconut oil to the liquid ingredients. Add the nuts and mix together. Combine the wet ingredients and the dry ingredients in one bowl and mix just until moist. Do not overmix or the muffins will not rise as well. Fill the muffin cups half full. Bake for 15 minutes, or until a toothpick inserted in the center comes out clean.   MAKES 12 MUFFINS

Blueberry-Coconut Muffins

Coconut oil, for greasing the muffin pan

1 cup (125 g) whole-wheat flour, plus more for dusting the muffin pan

½ cup (120 ml) coconut milk

1 large egg

½ cup (170 g) honey

1 teaspoon vanilla extract

½ cup (42 g) grated coconut

2 teaspoons baking powder

¼ teaspoon salt

1 cup (145 g) fresh blueberries

PREHEAT THE OVEN TO 400°F (200°C). Coat a muffin pan with a thin layer of coconut oil and dust with flour. In a medium bowl, combine the coconut milk, egg, honey, and vanilla and mix thoroughly. In a separate bowl, mix together the flour, coconut, baking powder, and salt. Add the dry ingredients to the wet ingredients, mixing just until moistened. Fold in the blueberries. Fill the muffin cups half full. Bake for 15 minutes, or until a toothpick inserted in the center comes out clean.   MAKES 12 MUFFINS

RASPBERRY-COCONUT MUFFINS

Follow the directions for making Blueberry-Coconut Muffins (above), substituting raspberries for the blueberries.

CHERRY-COCONUT MUFFINS

Follow the directions for making Blueberry-Coconut Muffins (above), substituting tart cherries for the blueberries.

Cinnamon-Nut Muffins

Coconut oil, for greasing the muffin pan

½ cup (62 g) flour, plus more for dusting the muffin pan

½ cup (120 ml) coconut milk

1 large egg

2 tablespoons (40 g) honey

1 teaspoon almond extract

1 teaspoon baking powder

½ teaspoon ground cinnamon

¼ teaspoon salt

¼ cup (28 g) pecans

2 tablespoons (11 g) grated coconut

PREHEAT THE OVEN TO 400°F (200°C). Coat a muffin pan with a thin layer of coconut oil and dust with flour. In a medium bowl, combine the coconut milk, egg, honey, and almond extract and mix thoroughly. In a separate bowl, mix together the flour, baking powder, cinnamon, and salt. Add the dry ingredients to the wet ingredients, mixing just until moistened. Fold in the pecans and coconut. Fill the muffin cups half full. Bake for 15 minutes, or until a toothpick inserted in the center comes out clean.   MAKES 6 MUFFINS

Corn Bread Muffins

Coconut oil, for greasing the muffin pan

¼ cup (31 g) flour, plus more for dusting the muffin pan

½ cup (120 ml) coconut milk

1 large egg

2 tablespoons (40 g) honey

1 teaspoon vanilla extract

¼ cup (35 g) cornmeal

1 teaspoon baking powder

¼ teaspoon salt

PREHEAT THE OVEN TO 400°F (200°C). Coat a muffin pan with a thin layer of coconut oil and dust with flour. In a medium bowl, combine the coconut milk, egg, honey, and vanilla and mix thoroughly. In a separate bowl, mix together the cornmeal, flour, baking powder, and salt. Add the dry ingredients to the wet ingredients, mixing just until moistened. Fill the muffin cups half full. Bake for 15 minutes, or until a toothpick inserted in the center comes out clean.   MAKES 6 MUFFINS

COCONUT–CORN BREAD MUFFINS

Make the Corn Bread Muffins (page 148) according to the directions and add 2 tablespoons (10.6 g) of grated coconut to the batter.   **MAKES 6 MUFFINS**

Whole-Wheat Coconut Pancakes

1 cup (125 g) whole-wheat flour
1½ teaspoons baking powder
¼ teaspoon salt
¼ cup (21 g) grated coconut
1 large egg
1 tablespoon (20 g) molasses (see Note)
2 tablespoons plus 2 teaspoons (40 ml) coconut oil, melted
1¼ cups (295 ml) lukewarm water

IN A MEDIUM BOWL, mix together the flour, baking powder, salt, and coconut. In a separate bowl, combine the egg, molasses, 2 tablespoons (30 ml) of the coconut oil, and the lukewarm water. Warm water is used to keep the coconut oil from hardening. In a large skillet, heat the remaining 2 teaspoons (10 ml) of coconut oil over medium heat. Mix the dry ingredients with the wet ingredients. Spoon the batter onto the hot skillet, making pancakes about 2½ to 3 inches (6.5 to 7.5 cm) in diameter. Serve with your choice of syrup, fruit, or Coconut Sauce (page 61).   **MAKES 8 TO 10 PANCAKES**

Note
Honey can be substituted for the molasses if desired.

Coconut Milk Pancakes

1 cup (125 g) flour
1 teaspoon baking powder
¼ teaspoon salt
1 large egg
1½ cups (355 ml) coconut milk
1 teaspoon vanilla extract
2 teaspoons (10 ml) coconut oil

IN A MEDIUM BOWL, mix the flour, baking powder, and salt. In a separate bowl, mix together the egg, coconut milk, and vanilla. Stir the dry ingredients into the wet ingredients. In a large skillet, heat the coconut oil over medium heat. Spoon the batter onto the hot skillet, making pancakes about 2½ to 3 inches (6.5 to 7.5 cm) in diameter. For thinner pancakes, add a little water. **MAKES ABOUT 8 PANCAKES**

Orange-Coconut Pancakes

> 1 cup (125 g) flour
> 1 teaspoon baking powder
> ¼ teaspoon salt
> 1 large egg
> ¾ cup (175 ml) coconut milk
> 6 tablespoons (90 ml) orange juice concentrate, no water added
> 2 teaspoons (10 ml) coconut oil

IN A MEDIUM BOWL, mix the flour, baking powder, and salt. In a separate bowl, combine the egg, coconut milk, and orange juice concentrate. Stir the dry ingredients into the wet ingredients. In a large skillet, heat the coconut oil over medium heat. Spoon the batter onto the hot skillet, making pancakes about 3 inches (7.5 cm) in diameter. Cook until puffed and dry around the edges. Turn and cook the other side. Serve with syrup or your favorite topping. **MAKES ABOUT 8 PANCAKES**

FRUITY COCONUT PANCAKES
Make the Orange-Coconut Pancakes (above) as directed, but substitute any variety of frozen fruit juice concentrates for the orange juice.
MAKES ABOUT 8 PANCAKES

Coconutty Pancakes

¾ cup (94 g) flour

½ cup (42 g) shredded coconut

⅓ cup (about 45 g) nuts

1 teaspoon baking powder

¼ teaspoon salt

2 large eggs

¾ cup (175 ml) coconut milk

½ cup (80 g) crushed fresh pineapple

2 teaspoons (10 ml) coconut oil

IN A MEDIUM BOWL, mix together the flour, coconut, nuts, baking powder, and salt. In a separate bowl, combine the eggs, coconut milk, and pineapple. Stir the dry ingredients into the wet ingredients. In a large skillet, heat the coconut oil over medium heat. Spoon the batter onto the hot skillet, making pancakes about 3 inches (7.5 cm) in diameter. Cook until puffed and dry around the edges. Turn and cook the other side. Serve with syrup or your favorite topping. **MAKES ABOUT 8 PANCAKES**

Coconut-Banana Pancakes

1 cup (235 ml) coconut milk

2 large eggs

½ teaspoon almond extract

1 cup (125 g) flour

½ cup (42 g) grated coconut

1 tablespoon (13 g) sugar

2 teaspoons baking powder

½ teaspoon salt

1 banana, sliced and quartered

2 teaspoons coconut oil

IN A MEDIUM BOWL, beat together the coconut milk, eggs, and almond extract. In a separate bowl, mix the flour, coconut, sugar, baking powder, and salt. Combine the wet ingredients and dry ingredients, mixing just until moistened. Fold the banana pieces into the batter. For thinner pancakes, add more coconut milk. In a large skillet, heat the coconut oil over medium heat. Drop the batter onto the hot skillet. Cook until small bubbles appear. Flip and cook the other side until done. Top with Coconut Sauce (page 61) or syrup.   MAKES ABOUT 10 PANCAKES

Baked Blueberry Pancake

2 tablespoons (¼ stick/28 g) salted butter

3 large eggs

1 can (14 ounces/400 ml) coconut milk

¾ cup (94 g) flour

2 tablespoons (26 g) sugar

½ teaspoon salt

½ teaspoon ground cinnamon

1 cup (145 g) blueberries

PREHEAT THE OVEN TO 425°F (220°C). Put the butter in a 10-inch (25-cm) pie plate and melt it in the oven. Be careful not to burn the butter. While the butter is melting, in a medium bowl, beat the eggs, coconut milk, flour, sugar, and salt until smooth. Pour the mixture into the hot pie plate. Bake for 20 minutes. Remove the pie plate from the oven and sprinkle the top with the cinnamon and blueberries. Bake for 10 to 15 minutes longer, or until a knife inserted in the center comes out clean and the pancake is browned and puffed. Serve hot. If a sweeter pancake is desired, top with a little honey or whipped cream.   SERVES 4

BAKED PEACH PANCAKE

Make the Baked Blueberry Pancake (above) recipe according to the directions, substituting 1 to 2 cups (170 to 340 g) of sliced peaches for the blueberries.

REDUCED-SUGAR BAKED BLUEBERRY PANCAKE

Make the Baked Blueberry Pancake (above) recipe according to directions, but omit the sugar and add a dash or two of stevia. Taste the batter for desired sweetness before cooking.

Crepes

1 cup (125 g) flour
1 teaspoon sugar
½ teaspoon baking powder
¼ teaspoon salt
2 large eggs
1 can (14 ounces/400 ml) coconut milk
2 tablespoons plus 2 teaspoons (40 ml) coconut oil, melted
1 teaspoon vanilla extract

IN A MEDIUM BOWL, mix together the flour, sugar, baking powder, and salt. Stir in the eggs, coconut milk, 2 tablespoons (30 ml) of the coconut oil, and the vanilla and beat until smooth. In a 6- to 8-inch (15- to 20-cm) skillet, heat the remaining 2 teaspoons (10 ml) of coconut oil over medium heat. Pour ¼ cup (60 ml) of the batter into the skillet; immediately rotate the skillet until a thin, even layer of batter covers the bottom of the pan. Cook for about 4 minutes, until the crepe is light golden brown and the edges begin to pull away from the surface of the pan. Run a pancake turner around the edge to loosen the crepe; then flip it over and cook the other side. Stack the crepes, placing wax paper between each layer. Keep them covered. To serve, cover one side of crepes with your choice of chopped fruit, nuts, jelly, and/or whipped cream. Roll up and sprinkle with confectioners' sugar.
MAKES ABOUT 8 CREPES

French Toast

2 large eggs
¼ cup (60 ml) coconut milk
1 teaspoon ground cinnamon
⅛ teaspoon salt
4 slices of bread
2 teaspoons (10 ml) coconut oil

IN A MEDIUM BOWL, beat the eggs, coconut milk, cinnamon, and salt together until smooth. Dip the bread in the egg mixture until completely covered. In a large skillet, melt the coconut oil over medium heat. Add the bread and cook for about 5 minutes on each side, until golden brown. Serve topped with fresh fruit or syrup.   SERVES 4

Scones ✿

> Coconut oil for deep-frying
> 1 cup (125 g) flour
> 1 teaspoon baking powder
> ½ teaspoon salt
> 2 large eggs
> 1 tablespoon (20 g) honey
> ¼ cup (60 ml) water
> 1 teaspoon vanilla extract

FILL A MEDIUM saucepan with coconut oil to a depth of ¾ inch (20 mm) and place over medium heat, or use a deep fryer. Heat the oil to about 325°F (170°C) on a deep-fry thermometer. In a medium bowl, mix together the flour, baking powder, and salt. In a separate bowl, thoroughly mix the eggs, honey, water, and vanilla. Add the dry ingredients to the wet ingredients and mix just until moist. Do not overmix. Drop the batter by the spoonful into the hot oil. Cook until the bottom side is lightly browned, then flip over. Each side should cook about a minute or so. Remove from the oil and place on a paper towel–lined plate to drain. Serve with confectioners' sugar and cinnamon, honey, jam, or syrup.   MAKES ABOUT 12 SCONES

Granola ✿

> 6 cups (480 g) old-fashioned oats
> 2 teaspoons ground cinnamon
> 4 cups (340 g) shredded or flaked coconut
> 2 cups (220 g) slivered or sliced almonds
> 1 cup (218 g) virgin coconut oil
> 1 cup (340 g) honey
> 1 tablespoon (15 ml) vanilla extract or almond extract
> Raisins, for serving (optional)
> Dried fruit, for serving (optional)

PREHEAT THE OVEN TO 325°F (170°C). In a large bowl, mix together the oats, cinnamon, coconut, and almonds. In a small saucepan, heat the coconut oil and honey over medium heat until hot; remove from the heat and add the vanilla. Stir the honey mixture into the oat mixture. Pour into a 15 x 10 x 1.5 inch (38 x 25 x 4 cm) baking pan. Bake for 1 hour and 15 minutes, or until golden brown. Stir occasionally while cooking, for even browning. Cool. Add the raisins or dried fruit if desired.   SERVES 8

REDUCED-SUGAR GRANOLA
Make the Granola (page 154) as directed, but replace the honey with 1 cup (345 g) of rice syrup. Add the raisins or dried fruit if more sweetening is desired.   SERVES 8

Coconut Oatmeal ✿

1¾ cups (410 ml) water
¼ teaspoon salt
½ cup (42 g) grated coconut
1 cup (80 g) old-fashioned oats
⅛ teaspoon almond extract

IN A MEDIUM SAUCEPAN, bring the water and salt to a rolling boil over moderately high heat. Add the coconut and oats. Reduce the heat to medium-low and simmer for 5 minutes. Remove from the heat, stir in the almond extract, cover, and let sit for 4 minutes. Add the sweetener of your choice and serve with any one of the following: milk, coconut milk, Sweetened Coconut Milk (page 21), Powerhouse Mango Milk (page 40), or any Fresh Fruit–Flavored Milks (page 22).   SERVES 2 TO 3

FRESH FRUIT COCONUT OATMEAL
Make the Coconut Oatmeal (above) as directed and add fresh fruit cut into bite-size pieces. This tastes good with peaches, nectarines, pineapple, mango, papaya, banana, strawberries, blueberries, kiwi, boysenberries, raspberries, or blackberries.

REDUCED-SUGAR COCONUT OATMEAL

Make the Coconut Oatmeal (above) as directed, and add fruit of your choice and sweeten with stevia to taste.

Coconut Rice

½ cup (95 g) brown rice

1½ cups (355 ml) water

1 cup (235 ml) coconut milk

1 teaspoon vanilla extract

2 tablespoons (40 g) sucanat or honey

¼ teaspoon salt

1 cup (85 g) shredded coconut, toasted

IN A MEDIUM SAUCEPAN, soak the rice in the water for 4 hours or overnight. Keep the rice covered as it soaks. Bring the rice and water to a boil over medium-high heat. Reduce the heat to medium-low, cover, and gently simmer for about 45 minutes, or until the water is absorbed. Remove from the heat. Mix in the coconut milk, vanilla, sucanat, and salt. Serve topped with toasted coconut.   SERVES 2

FRUIT COCONUT RICE

As a variation of Coconut Rice (above), you can add fresh cut-up fruit to the rice just before serving. Mangos, peaches, and strawberries make good accompaniments, but almost any fruit will work.

Indian-Style Coconut Rice

This is a mildly spicy rice dish that makes an excellent breakfast.

½ cup (95 g) brown rice

1½ cups (355 ml) water

½ cup (42 g) grated or shredded coconut

2 tablespoons (18 g) raisins

2 tablespoons (about 20 g) sucanat or other sweetener

¼ teaspoon ground cardamom

1 teaspoon ground cinnamon

¼ teaspoon salt

1 cup (235 ml) coconut milk

2 to 3 tablespoons (14 to 21 g) slivered almonds, toasted

IN A MEDIUM SAUCEPAN, soak the rice in the water for 4 hours or overnight. Keep the rice covered as it soaks. Bring the rice and water to a boil over medium-high heat. Add the coconut, raisins, sucanat, cardamom, cinnamon, and salt. Reduce the heat to medium-low, cover, and gently simmer for 45 minutes, or until the water is absorbed. Mix in the coconut milk. Remove from the heat. Serve topped with the toasted almonds.   SERVES 3 TO 4

REDUCED-SUGAR INDIAN-STYLE COCONUT RICE

Follow the directions for making Indian-Style Coconut Rice (page 156), but eliminate the sucanat, increase the raisins to ½ cup (75 g), and add stevia to taste. Fresh fruit may also be added.

Coconut Milk Biscuits ✿

1 large egg, at room temperature

½ cup (120 ml) coconut milk, at room temperature

2 tablespoons (30 ml) coconut oil, melted but not hot

1½ cups (188 g) flour

1½ teaspoons baking powder

½ teaspoon salt

PREHEAT THE OVEN TO 400°F (200°C). In a medium bowl, combine the egg, coconut milk, and coconut oil. In a separate bowl, mix together the flour, baking powder, and salt. Add the dry ingredients to the wet ingredients and mix just until moistened. Roll the dough into 1½-inch (4-cm) balls and place on an ungreased baking sheet. Flour your hands to keep the dough from sticking. Flatten each ball so that the dough is about ½ inch (13 mm) thick. Bake for 20 minutes.   MAKES 6 TO 8 BISCUITS

Cheese Biscuits ⚙

> 1 cup (125 g) flour, plus more to coat the biscuits
> 1 teaspoon baking powder
> ½ teaspoon salt
> 2 tablespoons (30 ml) coconut oil, melted
> ½ cup (120 ml) Thick Cheddar Cheese Sauce (page 63)
> 1 large egg
> 2 tablespoons (20 g) diced onions

PREHEAT THE OVEN TO 400°F (200°C). In a medium bowl, mix together the flour, baking powder, and salt. In a separate bowl, blend together the melted coconut oil with warm (not hot) Thick Cheddar Cheese Sauce. Stir in the egg and onion; the mixture will be lumpy. Add the flour mixture. The dough will be very soft at this stage. Shape into 1½-inch (4-cm) balls, roll in flour to coat, and place on an ungreased baking sheet. Bake for 12 to 15 minutes. MAKES 6 TO 8 BISCUITS

DOUBLE CHEESE BISCUITS

This recipe is for those who love cheese. Make the Cheese Biscuits (page 157) as directed, and add ½ cup (about 78 g) of shredded cheese to the batter.

Yorkshire Pudding ⚙

This delicious bread pudding is traditionally eaten with roast beef and smothered in gravy. Ordinarily Yorkshire Pudding is made with milk; this version, however, uses coconut milk.

> ¼ cup (55 g) meat drippings or unsalted butter
> 2 large eggs
> 1 cup (235 ml) coconut milk
> 1 cup (125 g) flour
> ½ teaspoon salt
> Gravy, for serving (pages 64–67)

PREHEAT THE OVEN TO 400°F (200°C). Coat the bottom of a 9 x 9 x 2-inch (23 x 23 x 5-cm) pan with the meat drippings. In the bowl of a blender, mix the eggs, coconut milk, flour, and salt at high speed for 1 to 2 minutes, until the mixture is bubbly. Pour the mixture into the prepared pan and bake for 20 minutes. Serve hot with gravy.   SERVES 8

Hush Puppies

Coconut oil for deep-frying

¾ cup (105 g) cornmeal

½ cup (62 g) flour, plus more to coat the hush puppies

1 teaspoon baking powder

¾ teaspoon salt

1 teaspoon onion powder

1 cup (235 ml) coconut milk

1 large egg

¼ cup (40 g) finely chopped onion

¼ cup (38 g) finely chopped red bell pepper

¼ cup (42 g) whole kernel corn

IN A LARGE SAUCEPAN, add coconut oil to a depth of 1.5 inches (4 cm). Heat the oil over medium heat to about 325°F (170°C) on a deep-fry thermometer. In a medium bowl, mix together the cornmeal, flour, baking powder, salt, and onion powder. Stir in the coconut milk and egg. Fold in the onion, bell pepper, and corn. Form the batter into 1-inch (2.5-cm) balls and roll in flour to coat. Drop the batter into the hot oil. Fry until brown, about 3 minutes. Remove to a paper towel–lined plate.   MAKES ABOUT 12 HUSH PUPPIES

Coconut-Banana Bread with Lime Glaze

Coconut oil for greasing the loaf pan

2 cups (250 g) flour, plus more for dusting the loaf pan

½ cup (42 g) grated coconut

2 teaspoons baking powder

1 cup (200 g) sucanat or sugar

½ teaspoon salt

½ cup (118 ml) coconut oil, melted

2 large eggs

1½ cups (338 g) mashed ripe banana (about 3 bananas)

1 teaspoon vanilla extract

Lime Glaze (recipe below)

PREHEAT THE OVEN TO 350°F (180°C). Coat an 8½ x 4½-inch (21.5 x 11.5-cm) loaf pan with a thin layer of coconut oil and dust with flour. In a large bowl, combine the flour, coconut, baking powder, sucanat, and salt. In a separate bowl, blend the coconut oil and eggs; mix in the banana and vanilla. Combine the wet ingredients and the dry ingredients and mix just until moist. Pour the batter into the prepared loaf pan. Bake for 55 to 60 minutes, or until a knife inserted in the center comes out clean. Cool the loaf in the pan for 10 minutes on a wire rack. Remove from the pan and let cool completely on the wire rack. Pour Lime Glaze over top.   MAKES 1 LOAF

Lime Glaze

½ cup (60 g) confectioners' sugar

1½ tablespoons (25 ml) freshly squeezed lime juice or lemon
   juice

BLEND THE CONFECTIONERS' sugar and lime juice. Drizzle over the warm banana bread.   MAKES ⅓ CUP

REDUCED-SUGAR COCONUT-BANANA BREAD

Make the Coconut-Banana Bread with Lime Glaze (page 159) as directed, but reduce the sucanat to ⅓ cup (69 g) and add ¼ teaspoon of stevia. Omit the glaze.

Hawaiian Banana Bread

Coconut oil, to coat the loaf pan

2 cups (250 g) flour, plus more for dusting the loaf pan

½ cup (42 g) grated coconut

2 teaspoons baking powder

1 cup (200 g) sucanat or sugar

½ teaspoon salt

½ cup (118 ml) coconut oil, melted

2 large eggs

1 ripe banana, mashed

1 can (8 ounces/226 g) crushed pineapple with juice

¼ cup (71 g) orange juice concentrate, no water added

PREHEAT THE OVEN TO 350°F (180°C). Coat an 8½ x 4½-inch (21.5 x 11.5-cm) loaf pan with a thin layer of coconut oil and dust with flour. In a large bowl, combine the flour, coconut, baking powder, sucanat, and salt. In a separate bowl, blend the coconut oil and eggs; mix in the banana, pineapple, and orange juice concentrate. Combine the wet ingredients and the dry ingredients and mix just until moist. Pour the batter into the prepared loaf pan and bake for 55 to 60 minutes, or until a knife inserted in the center comes out clean. Cool the loaf in the pan for 10 minutes on a wire rack. Remove from the pan and let cool completely on the wire rack.

MAKES 1 LOAF

REDUCED-SUGAR HAWAIIAN BANANA BREAD

Make Hawaiian Banana Bread (above) as directed, but reduce the sucanat to ⅓ cup (69 g) and add ¼ teaspoon of stevia. MAKES 1 LOAF

Orange-Coconut Banana Bread

Coconut oil to coat the loaf pan

1½ cups (188 g) flour, plus more for dusting the loaf pan

½ cup (42 g) grated coconut

⅓ cup (40 g) chopped walnuts

¾ teaspoon baking powder

¾ cup (150 g) sucanat or sugar

½ teaspoon salt

¼ cup (60 ml) coconut milk

2 large eggs

1½ cups (338 g) mashed ripe banana (about 3 bananas)

1½ tablespoons (9 g) grated orange rind

¼ cup (71 g) orange juice concentrate, no water added

PREHEAT THE OVEN TO 350°F (180°C). Coat an 8½ x 4½-inch (21.5 x 11.5-cm) loaf pan with a thin layer of coconut oil and dust with flour. In a large bowl, combine the flour, coconut, walnuts, baking powder, sucanat, and salt. In a separate bowl, mix together the coconut milk, eggs, banana, orange rind, and orange juice concentrate. Combine the wet ingredients and the dry ingredients and mix just until moist. Pour the batter into the prepared loaf pan. Bake for 55 to 60 minutes, or until a knife inserted in the center comes out clean. Cool the loaf in the pan for 10 minutes on a wire rack. Remove from the pan and let cool completely on the wire rack.

MAKES 1 LOAF

REDUCED-SUGAR ORANGE COCONUT BANANA BREAD

Make the Orange-Coconut Banana Bread (page 161) as directed, but reduce the sucanat to ⅓ cup (69 g) and add ¼ teaspoon stevia.

Pumpkin-Nut Bread

Coconut oil to coat the loaf pan

1¼ cups (156 g) flour, plus more for dusting the loaf pan

½ cup (42 g) grated coconut

½ cup (about 55 g) chopped nuts

1 teaspoon baking powder

½ teaspoon baking soda

¾ cup (150 g) sucanat or sugar

1 teaspoon ground cinnamon

½ teaspoon ground nutmeg

1 teaspoon salt

1 cup (235 ml) coconut milk

2 large eggs

1 cup (245 g) canned pumpkin puree

PREHEAT THE OVEN TO 350°F (180°C). Coat an 8½ x 4½-inch (21.5 x 11.5-cm) loaf pan with a thin layer of coconut oil and dust with flour. In a large bowl, combine the flour, coconut, nuts, baking powder, baking soda, sucanat, cinnamon, nutmeg, and salt. In a separate bowl, blend together the coconut milk, eggs, and pumpkin. Combine the wet ingredients and the dry ingredients and mix just until moist. Pour the batter into the prepared loaf pan. Bake for 60 to 65 minutes, or until a knife inserted in the center comes out clean. Cool the loaf in the pan for 10 minutes on a wire rack. Remove from the pan and let cool completely on the wire rack.   MAKES 1 LOAF

REDUCED-SUGAR PUMPKIN-NUT BREAD

Make the Pumpkin-Nut Bread (page 162) as directed, but reduce the sucanat to ⅓ cup (69 g) and add ¼ teaspoon of stevia.

CAKES

Coconut Cake

Coconut oil for greasing the baking pan

1 cup (125 g) whole-wheat flour, plus more for dusting the baking pan

1 cup (235 ml) coconut milk

1 cup (200 g) sugar

½ teaspoon vanilla extract

¼ teaspoon almond extract

2 large eggs

2 teaspoons baking powder

¼ teaspoon salt

Coconut Frosting (page 166)

PREHEAT THE OVEN TO 350°F (180°C). Coat an 11 x 7 x 2-inch (30 x 18 x 5-cm) baking pan with a thin layer of coconut oil and dust with flour. In a medium bowl, stir together the coconut milk, sugar, vanilla, almond extract, and eggs. In a separate bowl, sift together the flour, baking powder, and salt. Stir the dry ingredients into the wet ingredients. Pour the batter into the prepared baking pan. Bake for about 25 minutes, or until light golden brown and the cake begins to pull away from the sides of the pan. Cool for about 15 minutes and top with Coconut Frosting. SERVES 8

Coconut Frosting

> 2 tablespoons (30 ml) coconut oil, melted
> ¼ cup (60 ml) coconut milk
> 2 cups (240 g) confectioners' sugar
> 1 teaspoon vanilla extract
> ⅛ teaspoon salt
> ½ cup (42 g) shredded coconut, toasted

IN A MEDIUM BOWL, cream together the coconut oil, coconut milk, confectioners' sugar, vanilla, and salt. Spread on the completely cooled cake and sprinkle the top with toasted coconut.   MAKES 1 CUP FROSTING

German Chocolate Cake ✿

This cake is made with Dutch cocoa, which is very popular in Europe. Dutching is a process that neutralizes the natural acidity in cocoa powder, producing a chocolate with less bitter flavor. Regular cocoa can be substituted for Dutch process cocoa if you like. The recipe below makes a single layer sheet cake or two layers of a 9-inch (23-cm) layer cake.

> Coconut oil for greasing the baking pan
> 2½ cups (312 g) flour, plus more for dusting the baking pan
> ⅔ cup (150 g) salted butter
> ⅔ cup (57 g) Dutch cocoa
> 1 cup (235 ml) coconut milk
> 1¾ cups (350 g) sugar
> 1 teaspoon vanilla extract
> 4 large eggs, separated
> 2 teaspoons baking powder
> ½ teaspoon salt
> ⅛ teaspoon cream of tartar
> Coconut-Pecan Frosting (page 167)

PREHEAT THE OVEN TO 350°F (180°C). Coat a 13 x 9 x 2-inch (33 x 23 x 5-cm) baking pan with a thin layer of coconut oil and dust with flour. In a small saucepan, melt the butter and cocoa over low heat. Stir until smooth, remove from the heat, and let cool slightly. Stir in the coconut milk, sugar, vanilla, and egg yolks. In a medium bowl, mix together the flour, baking powder, and salt. Stir the dry ingredients into the chocolate mixture. In the bowl of a standing mixer, beat the egg whites and cream of tartar at high speed until soft peaks form. Fold the egg whites into the batter. Pour the batter into the prepared baking pan. Bake for 35 to 40 minutes, or until a knife inserted in the center comes out clean. If you want to make a layer cake, use 2 round 9-inch (23-cm) pans and bake for about 30 minutes. Remove from the oven and let cool. Cover the top of the cake with Coconut-Pecan Frosting.   SERVES 15

Coconut-Pecan Frosting

This recipe makes enough frosting to frost only the top of the cake. If you want to frost the sides as well, double the recipe.

> ½ cup (120 ml) coconut milk
> 2 teaspoons cornstarch
> ½ cup (100 g) sugar
> 1 large egg yolk (see Note)
> ¼ cup (½ stick/55 g) salted butter
> ½ teaspoon vanilla extract
> ¾ cup (64 g) flaked coconut
> ½ cup (55 g) chopped pecans

IN A SMALL SAUCEPAN, mix together the coconut milk, cornstarch, sugar, egg yolk, and butter. Cook over medium heat, stirring constantly, for 5 to 6 minutes, until the mixture thickens. Remove from the heat and add the vanilla, coconut, and pecans.   MAKES ABOUT 2 CUPS (475 ML)

Note

The frosting does not use the egg white. However, you can make use of it by combining it with the egg whites used in the batter recipe.

REDUCED-SUGAR GERMAN CHOCOLATE CAKE

Make the German Chocolate Cake (page 166) as directed, but reduce the sugar to ¾ to 1 cup (150 to 200 g) and add 1 tablespoon (8 g) of flour and ¼ teaspoon of stevia. Make the frosting as directed, but reduce the sugar to ¼ cup (50 g).   SERVES 12

Banana-Coconut Cake

1 cup (240 ml) coconut oil, melted, plus more for greasing the
   baking pan
2⅓ cups (292 g) flour, plus more for dusting the baking pan
1⅔ cups (333 g) sugar
1¼ teaspoons baking powder
1 teaspoon baking soda
1 teaspoon salt
2 large eggs
1½ cups (338 g) mashed ripe bananas (about 2 bananas)
2 teaspoons freshly squeezed lemon juice
¾ cup (64 g) shredded coconut

PREHEAT THE OVEN TO 350°F (180°C). Coat a 13 x 9 x 2-inch (33 x 23 x 5-cm) baking pan with a thin layer of coconut oil and dust with flour. In a large bowl, mix together the flour, sugar, baking powder, baking soda, and salt. Add the coconut oil, eggs, banana, and lemon juice and mix until all of the flour is dampened. Beat vigorously for 2 minutes. Fold in the coconut. Pour the batter into the prepared baking pan and bake for 35 minutes, or until a knife inserted in the center comes out clean. Cool for 10 minutes in the pan.   SERVES 12

REDUCED-SUGAR BANANA-COCONUT CAKE
Make the Banana-Coconut Cake (above) as directed, but reduce the sugar to ¾ cup (150 g), add ⅛ teaspoon of stevia, and reduce the coconut oil to ½ cup (120 ml).

Applesauce Cake

½ cup (120 ml) coconut oil, melted, plus more for greasing
   the baking pan
2½ cups (312 g) flour, plus more for dusting the baking pan
1½ teaspoons baking soda
1 teaspoon salt
1 teaspoon ground cinnamon

½ teaspoon ground nutmeg

¼ teaspoon ground allspice

2 large eggs

2 cups (400 g) sugar

1½ cups (380 g) applesauce

½ cup (55 g) chopped pecans

PREHEAT THE OVEN TO 350°F (180°C). Coat a 13 x 9 x 2-inch (33 x 23 x 5-cm) baking pan with a layer of coconut oil and dust with flour. In a medium bowl, combine the flour, baking soda, salt, cinnamon, nutmeg, and allspice. Set aside. In a separate bowl, blend together the eggs and coconut oil. Add in the sugar and applesauce. Stir in the flour mixture. Fold in the pecans. Pour the batter into the prepared baking pan and bake for about 40 minutes, or until a knife inserted in the center comes out clean. Cool for 10 minutes in the pan.   SERVES 12

REDUCED-SUGAR APPLESAUCE CAKE

Follow the directions for making the Applesauce Cake (page 168), but reduce the sugar to 1 cup (200 g), add ⅛ teaspoon of stevia, and reduce the applesauce to 1 cup (245 g).

Coconut-Carrot Cake

1½ cups (360 ml) coconut oil, melted, plus more for greasing the baking pan

2 cups (250 g) flour, plus more for dusting the baking pan

2 teaspoons baking soda

2 teaspoons ground cinnamon

½ teaspoon ground nutmeg

3 large eggs

1½ cups (300 g) sucanat or sugar

1 teaspoon vanilla extract

1 can (8 ounces/226 g) crushed pineapple

2 cups (220 g) grated carrots

1 cup (110 g) chopped pecans

1 cup (85 g) grated coconut

PREHEAT THE OVEN TO 350°F (180°C). Coat a 13 x 9 x 2-inch (33 x 23 x 5-cm) baking pan with a layer of coconut oil and dust with flour. In a medium bowl, mix together the flour, baking soda, cinnamon, and nutmeg; set aside. In a separate bowl, beat together the eggs and the melted (but not hot) coconut oil; mix in the sucanat, vanilla, and pineapple. Combine the dry ingredients and the wet ingredients. Add the carrots, pecans, and coconut. Pour the batter into the prepared baking pan and bake for 35 to 40 minutes, or until a knife inserted in the center comes out clean. Cool for about 15 minutes and top with your favorite frosting.   SERVES 12

REDUCED-SUGAR COCONUT-CARROT CAKE

Follow the directions for making the Coconut-Carrot Cake (page 169), but reduce the coconut oil to 1 cup (240 ml), reduce the sucanat to ¾ cup (150 g), and add ⅛ teaspoon of stevia.

Streusel Coconut Cake ⚙

Coconut oil, for greasing the baking pan
2 cups (250 g) flour, plus more for dusting the baking pan
1½ cups (300 g) sucanat or sugar
3 teaspoons baking powder
1 teaspoon salt
⅓ cup (75 g) salted butter
1 cup (235 ml) coconut milk
4 large eggs, slightly beaten
Streusel (recipe below)

PREHEAT THE OVEN TO 350°F (180°C). Coat a 13 x 9 x 2-inch (33 x 23 x 5-cm) baking pan with a layer of coconut oil and dust with flour. In a large bowl, mix the flour, sucanat, baking powder, and salt together. Add the butter, coconut milk, and eggs and stir until well blended. Pour the batter into the prepared baking pan. Cover the top with Streusel. Bake for 35 to 40 minutes, or until a knife inserted in the center comes out clean. Cool for about 10 minutes before serving.   SERVES 12

Streusel

½ cup (55 g) chopped pecans

½ cup (42 g) flaked or shredded coconut

⅓ cup (75 g) sucanat or firmly packed dark brown sugar

¼ cup (31 g) flour

1 teaspoon ground cinnamon

3 tablespoons (42 g) salted butter, softened

IN A MEDIUM MIXING BOWL, stir together the pecans, coconut, sucanat, flour, cinnamon, and butter. The streusel will have a crumbly texture.

MAKES ABOUT 1 CUP

PINEAPPLE-COCONUT CAKE

Make the Streusel Coconut Cake (page 170) as directed, but substitute ¼ cup (71 g) of frozen orange juice concentrate (thawed) for ¼ cup (60 ml) of the coconut milk. Add to the batter 1 can (8 ounces/226 g) of crushed pineapple, drained.

BLUEBERRY-COCONUT CAKE

Make the Streusel Coconut Cake (page 170) as directed, and add 1 cup (145 g) of blueberries to the batter.

APPLE-COCONUT CAKE

Peel and thinly slice 2 medium tart apples. Make the Streusel Coconut Cake (page 170) as directed, and add the apples to the batter.

REDUCED-SUGAR STREUSEL COCONUT CAKE

Make the Streusel Coconut Cake (page 170) as directed, but reduce the sucanat to ¾ cup (150 g) and add ¼ teaspoon of stevia. Follow the directions for the Streusel (above), reducing the sucanat to 1 tablespoon (13 g). Spread 1 cup or 1 can (8 ounces/227 g) of crushed pineapple, well drained, over the top.

Sponge Cake ✿

    Coconut oil, for greasing the baking pan

    2 cups (250 g) flour, plus more for dusting the baking pan

    7 large eggs, separated

    ½ teaspoon cream of tartar

    1½ cups (300 g) sugar

    1 tablespoon (16 g) baking powder

    ½ teaspoon salt

    1¼ cups (295 ml) coconut milk

    1 teaspoon vanilla extract

    Lemon Glaze (recipe below)

PREHEAT THE OVEN TO 350°F (180°C). Coat a 13 x 9 x 2-inch (33 x 23 x 5-cm) baking pan with a layer of coconut oil and dust with flour. In the bowl of a standing mixer, beat the egg whites and cream of tartar at high speed for about 3 minutes, until stiff peaks form; set aside. In a large mixing bowl, combine the flour, sugar, baking powder, and salt. Add the coconut milk, egg yolks, and vanilla and mix with an electric beater for about 4 minutes, until very smooth. Gradually and gently fold the batter into the egg whites with a rubber spatula, blending well. Pour the batter into the prepared baking pan and bake for about 35 minutes, or until the top springs back when lightly touched. Remove from the pan and let cool on a wire rack. Frost with Lemon Glaze. SERVES 12

VARIATION

If desired, this cake can be made using a 10-inch (25-cm) tube pan. Follow the recipe as directed, but increase the cooking time to 55 to 60 minutes. When the cake is removed from the oven, immediately invert it onto a funnel and let it hang upside down until completely cool. To remove the cake from the pan, run a knife around the outer edge of pan as well as around the tube. Remove from the pan and glaze.

Lemon Glaze

    2 cups (240 g) confectioners' sugar

    1 teaspoon vanilla extract

2 tablespoons (30 ml) freshly squeezed lemon juice

1 tablespoon (15 ml) coconut milk, or more for spreading consistency

2 teaspoons grated lemon peel

IN A MEDIUM BOWL, blend together the confectioners' sugar, vanilla, lemon juice, coconut milk, and lemon peel. Add more coconut milk as necessary to achieve the desired spreading consistency. Spread the glaze on the cooled cake. MAKES ABOUT 1 CUP

REDUCED-SUGAR SPONGE CAKE

Make the Sponge Cake (page 172) as directed, but reduce the sugar to ¾ cup (150 g) and add ⅛ teaspoon of stevia. Serve with Reduced-Sugar Coconut Whipped Cream (page 196).

Coconut Cream Cake

THIS IS A LAYER CAKE using the Sponge Cake recipe and a cream filling. Follow the directions for making the Sponge Cake batter (page 172). Bake in two greased 9-inch (23-cm) layer cake pans at 350°F (180°C) for 20 to 25 minutes, until the cakes shrink slightly from the sides of the pans and are springy to the touch. Cool upright in the pans on wire racks for 5 minutes, then remove from the pans and allow to cool completely. Fill and frost with one of the fillings below.

Basic Vanilla Cream Filling

¾ cup (175 ml) coconut milk

2 tablespoons (16 g) cornstarch

⅓ cup (69 g) sugar

1 large egg yolk, slightly beaten with ¼ cup coconut milk

1 teaspoon vanilla extract

½ teaspoon imitation coconut extract (optional)

IN A SMALL SAUCEPAN, mix together the coconut milk, cornstarch, and sugar. Bring to a boil over medium heat, stirring constantly, until the mixture thickens. Then boil and stir for ½ minute longer. Remove from the heat.

Slowly beat half of the hot mixture into the egg yolk, then gradually return all to the pan, beating constantly. Mix in the vanilla and the coconut extract, if using, and cool to room temperature.   MAKES ABOUT 1 CUP (235 ML), ENOUGH TO FILL AN 8- OR 9-INCH (20- OR 23-CM) 2-LAYER CAKE

COCONUT CREAM CAKE FILLING

Make a double recipe of the Basic Vanilla Cream Filling (page 173); divide in half and mix ½ cup (42 g) of flaked or shredded coconut into one part. Spread the coconut filling on one cake layer. Place the second cake layer on top. Spread the remaining filling over the top and sides of the cake, then coat thickly with flaked coconut (about 1½ cups/128 g).

CHOCOLATE-COCONUT CREAM FILLING

Prepare the Basic Vanilla Cream Filling (page 173) as directed, but add ½ cup (88 g) of semisweet chocolate chips along with the vanilla; blend well. Top with ½ cup (42 g) flaked or shredded coconut.

CITRUS CREAM FILLING

Prepare the Basic Vanilla Cream Filling (page 173) as directed, but omit the vanilla and add ¼ teaspoon of lemon or orange extract and 2 teaspoons of finely grated lemon or orange rind. Mix in ½ cup (42 g) of flaked or shredded coconut.

Strawberry Shortcake

THE SHORTCAKE in this recipe is actually a sponge cake. A muffin pan is used so they look like cupcakes. Even with whole-wheat flour, this recipe makes an incredibly light and tasty cake.

Coconut oil, for greasing the muffin pan
1 cup (125 g) flour, plus more for dusting the muffin pan
1½ teaspoons (3 g) baking powder
½ teaspoon salt
2 large eggs, separated
½ cup (120 ml) coconut milk
¼ cup (85 g) honey
1 teaspoon vanilla extract

⅛ teaspoon cream of tartar

3 to 4 cups (510 to 680 g) sliced strawberries

Coconut Whipped Cream (page 196)

PREHEAT THE OVEN TO 400°F (200°C). Coat a 12-cup muffin pan with a thin layer of coconut oil and dust with flour. In a medium mixing bowl, combine the flour, baking powder, and salt. In another bowl, blend together the egg yolks, coconut milk, honey, and vanilla. In the bowl of a standing mixer, beat the egg whites and cream of tartar at high speed for about 5 minutes, until soft peaks form. Stir the dry ingredients into the egg yolk mixture. Fold the egg whites into the batter just until blended; do not overmix. Pour the batter into the prepared muffin pan, filling the cups half full. Bake for 15 minutes. Cut the cakes in half and top each half with fresh sliced strawberries and Coconut Whipped Cream.   MAKES 24 SHORTCAKES

GINGER-PEACH SHORTCAKE

Make the shortcakes as directed in Strawberry Shortcake (page 174), but add ¼ cup (24 g) of chopped crystallized ginger to the batter. Top with sliced peaches and Coconut Whipped Cream (page 196).

REDUCED-SUGAR SHORTCAKES

Make shortcakes as directed in Strawberry Shortcake (page 174), but reduce the honey to 2 tablespoons (40 g) and add a dash of stevia. Use Reduced-Sugar Coconut Whipped Cream (page 196) with fresh strawberries for the topping.

Cinnamon-Apple Coconut Cake

1 cup (240 ml) coconut oil, melted, plus more for greasing the baking pan

2½ cups (312 g) flour, plus more for dusting the baking pan

1¾ cups (350 g) sucanat or sugar

2 teaspoons baking soda

1 teaspoon salt

4 large eggs, slightly beaten

2 teaspoons vanilla extract

2 teaspoons ground cinnamon

3 cups (375 g) cored, peeled, and chopped tart apples

2 cups (220 g) chopped pecans

½ cup (42 g) grated or shredded coconut

Coconut Whipped Cream (page 196)

PREHEAT THE OVEN TO 350°F (180°C). Coat a 13 x 9 x 2-inch (33 x 23 x 5-cm) baking pan with a thin layer of coconut oil and dust with flour. In a medium bowl, combine the flour, sucanat, baking soda, and salt. Mix in the melted (not hot) coconut oil, eggs, and vanilla. The batter will be stiff. In a separate bowl, mix together the cinnamon, apples, pecans, and coconut and fold the mixture into the batter. Pour the batter into the prepared baking pan and bake for 40 to 45 minutes, or until a knife inserted in the center comes out clean. Cool in the pan for 10 minutes. Serve topped with Coconut Whipped Cream. SERVES 12

REDUCED-SUGAR CINNAMON-APPLE COCONUT CAKE

Follow the directions for the Cinnamon-Apple Coconut Cake (page 175), but reduce the sucanat to ½ cup (100 g) and add ⅛ teaspoon of stevia.

COOKIES

Coconut Macaroons

> Coconut oil or coconut oil–based nonstick cooking spray, to coat the
>   baking sheet
> 2 large egg whites
> Dash of salt
> ½ teaspoon vanilla extract
> ⅔ cup (133 g) sugar
> 1 cup (85 g) shredded coconut

PREHEAT THE OVEN TO 325°F (170°C). Coat a baking sheet with a thin layer of coconut oil or nonstick cooking spray. In the bowl of a standing mixer, beat the egg whites with the salt and vanilla at high speed for about 4 minutes, until soft peaks form. Gradually add the sugar, beating until stiff. Fold in the coconut. Drop the batter by the rounded teaspoonful about 2 inches (5 cm) apart onto the prepared baking sheet. Bake for 20 minutes. While still hot, remove the cookies from the baking sheet and cool them on a wire rack. MAKES ABOUT 18 MACAROONS

PECAN MACAROONS
Follow the directions for making Coconut Macaroons (above), reducing the coconut to ¾ cup (64 g) and adding ½ cup (55 g) of chopped pecans.
MAKES ABOUT 18 MACAROONS

COCONUT-ALMOND MACAROONS

Follow the directions for making Coconut Macaroons (page 177), but substitute ½ teaspoon of almond extract for the vanilla. Reduce the coconut to ¾ cup (64 g) and add ½ cup (55 g) of slivered almonds.

CHOCOLATE MACAROONS

Follow the directions for making Coconut Macaroons (page 177), but add 1 tablespoon (11 g) of milk chocolate chips.

PINEAPPLE MACAROONS

Put ½ cup (85 g) of crushed or chopped pineapple on a paper towel and pat out the excess moisture. Follow the directions for making Coconut Macaroons (page 177), adding the pineapple to the mixture.

REDUCED-SUGAR MACAROONS

Make the Coconut Macaroons (page 177) according to the recipe, but reduce the sugar to ¼ cup (50 g) and add a dash or two of stevia. You can make any of the macaroon variations described above using this procedure.

Coconut Kisses

These cookies are similar to macaroons but with a crispy crunch.

> Coconut oil or coconut oil–based nonstick cooking spray, to coat the baking sheet
> 3 large egg whites
> ½ teaspoon vanilla extract
> Dash of salt
> ¾ cup (150 g) sugar
> 2 cups (56 g) crisp rice cereal
> 1 cup (85 g) shredded or grated coconut
> ½ cup (55 or 68 g) chopped almonds or macadamia nuts

PREHEAT THE OVEN TO 350°F (180°C). Coat a baking sheet with a thin layer of coconut oil or nonstick cooking spray. In the bowl of a standing mixer, beat the egg whites, vanilla, and salt at high speed for about 4 minutes, until soft peaks form. Gradually add the sugar, beating until stiff peaks form. Fold in the cereal, coconut, and nuts. Drop the batter by the teaspoonful about 2 inches (5 cm) apart onto the prepared baking sheet. Bake for 15 to 18 minutes, until lightly browned. Remove the cookies from the pan immediately and let cool on a wire rack. If they stick to the pan, reheat them in the oven to soften them. **MAKES ABOUT 2 DOZEN KISSES**

REDUCED-SUGAR COCONUT KISSES
Make Coconut Kisses (page 178) as directed but reduce sugar to ¼ cup (50 g) and add a dash or two of stevia.

Nutty Chocolate Chip Cookies ✿

> ½ cup (1 stick/112 g) salted butter
> ½ cup (115 g) sucanat or firmly packed dark brown sugar
> 1 large egg
> 1 teaspoon vanilla extract
> 1¼ cups (156 g) flour
> ½ cup (42 g) grated coconut
> ½ teaspoon salt
> ½ teaspoon baking powder
> ½ cup (88 g) semisweet chocolate chips
> ½ cup (55 g) chopped pecans

PREHEAT THE OVEN TO 375°F (190°C). In a medium bowl, combine the butter, sucanat, egg, and vanilla. In a separate bowl, mix together the flour, coconut, salt, and baking powder; blend into the egg mixture. Add the chocolate chips and pecans. Drop the dough by the teaspoonful about 2 inches (5 cm) apart onto an ungreased baking sheet. Bake for 10 to 12 minutes, until lightly browned. Remove from the baking sheet immediately and cool on a wire rack. **MAKES ABOUT 3 DOZEN COOKIES**

REDUCED-SUGAR NUTTY CHOCOLATE CHIP COOKIES
Make the Nutty Chocolate Chip Cookies (above) according to the directions, but reduce the sucanat to ¼ cup (60 g) and add a dash or two of stevia.

Coconut Meringue Bars

Coconut oil or coconut oil–based nonstick cooking spray,
   to coat the baking pan
¾ cup (1½ sticks/167 g) salted butter
3 large eggs, separated
½ cup (115 g) sucanat or firmly packed dark brown sugar
½ teaspoon vanilla extract
2 cups (250 g) flour
1 teaspoon baking powder
1 teaspoon baking soda
¼ teaspoon salt
1 cup (175 g) semisweet chocolate chips
1 cup (85 g) flaked coconut
1 cup (about 120 g) coarsely chopped nuts
¼ cup (100 g) granulated sugar
½ cup (42 g) grated coconut

PREHEAT THE OVEN TO 350°F (180°C). Coat a 13 x 9 x 2-inch (33 x 23 x 5-cm) baking pan with a thin layer of coconut oil or nonstick cooking spray. In a medium bowl, blend together the butter, egg yolks, sucanat, and vanilla; set aside. In a separate bowl, mix the flour, baking powder, baking soda, and salt. Mix together the wet ingredients and the dry ingredients. Fold in the chocolate chips, coconut, and nuts. Press the batter into the prepared baking pan.

In the bowl of a standing mixer, beat the egg whites at high speed for about 4 minutes, until foamy. Continue beating while adding the granulated sugar, 1 tablespoon (13 g) at a time; beat until stiff peaks form. Beat in the grated coconut. Spread over the mixture in the pan. Bake for 35 to 40 minutes, until golden brown. Cool.   MAKES 16 BARS

REDUCED-SUGAR COCONUT MERINGUE BARS
Make the Coconut Meringue Bars (page 180) as directed, but reduce the sucanat to ¼ cup (60 g) and add a dash or two of stevia. Reduce the sugar in the meringue to ¼ cup (50 g).

Carrot-Coconut Cookies

1 cup (338 g) mashed cooked carrot
¾ cup (150 g) sugar
1 cup (2 sticks/224 g) salted butter or coconut oil, melted
2 large eggs
2 cups (250 g) flour
2 teaspoons baking powder
½ teaspoon salt
¾ cup (64 g) shredded or flaked coconut
Orange Butter Frosting (recipe below)

PREHEAT THE OVEN TO 400°F (200°C). In a medium bowl, mix the carrot, sugar, butter, and eggs. Stir in the flour, baking powder, and salt. Stir in the coconut. Drop the dough by the teaspoonful about 2 inches (5 cm) apart onto an ungreased baking sheet. Bake for 8 minutes, or until almost no indentation remains when touched. Immediately remove the cookies from the baking sheet; cool on a wire rack, and frost with Orange Butter Frosting.
MAKES ABOUT 3 DOZEN COOKIES

Orange Butter Frosting

1½ cups (180 g) confectioners' sugar
¼ cup (½ stick/55 g) unsalted butter
2 tablespoons (30 ml) freshly squeezed orange juice
1 tablespoon (6 g) grated orange peel

MIX TOGETHER the confectioners' sugar and butter. Stir in the orange juice and orange peel; beat until the frosting is smooth. MAKES ABOUT 1 CUP

REDUCED-SUGAR CARROT-COCONUT COOKIES

Make the batter for the Carrot-Coconut Cookies (page 181) as directed, but reduce the sugar to ¼ cup (50 g) and add ⅛ teaspoon of stevia. Reduce the confectioners' sugar in the Orange Butter Frosting to 1 cup (120 g), add a dash of stevia, and reduce the butter to 3 tablespoons (42 g).

Coconut-Oatmeal Cookies

1 cup (225 g) firmly packed dark brown sugar

½ cup (1 stick/112 g) salted butter or coconut oil, melted

1 large egg

½ teaspoon vanilla extract

1 cup (125 g) flour

1 cup (80 g) quick-cooking or old-fashioned oats

½ cup (42 g) flaked coconut

½ teaspoon baking soda

¼ teaspoon salt

1½ teaspoons ground cinnamon

½ teaspoon ground nutmeg

½ cup (60 g) chopped walnuts

PREHEAT THE OVEN TO 375°F (190°C). In a medium bowl, mix together the brown sugar, butter, egg, and vanilla. In a separate bowl, combine the flour, oats, coconut, baking soda, salt, cinnamon, and nutmeg. Stir the dry ingredients into the wet mixture. Fold in the nuts. Drop the dough by the teaspoonful about 3 inches (8 cm) apart onto an ungreased baking sheet. Bake for 10 minutes. Remove the cookies from the baking sheet and let them cool on a wire rack.   MAKES ABOUT 2 DOZEN COOKIES

REDUCED-SUGAR COCONUT-OATMEAL COOKIES
Make the Coconut-Oatmeal Cookies (above) as described, but reduce the brown sugar to ½ cup (115 g) and add a dash or two of stevia. If desired, you can leave out the stevia and add ½ cup (75 g) of raisins.

Chocolate–Coconut-Oatmeal Cookies

1 cup (225 g) firmly packed dark brown sugar

½ cup (1 stick/112 g) salted butter, softened or melted

1 large egg

½ teaspoon vanilla extract

1 cup (125 g) flour

1 cup (80 g) quick-cooking or old-fashioned oats

½ cup (42 g) flaked coconut

½ teaspoon baking soda

¼ teaspoon salt

½ cup (55 g) chopped pecans

½ cup (88 g) semisweet chocolate chips

PREHEAT THE OVEN TO 375°F (190°C). In a medium bowl, combine the brown sugar, butter, egg, and vanilla. In a separate bowl, mix together the flour, oats, coconut, baking soda, and salt; stir into the wet mixture. Fold in the nuts and chocolate chips. Drop the dough by the teaspoonful about 3 inches (8 cm) apart onto an ungreased baking sheet. Bake for 10 minutes. Remove the cookies from the baking sheet and let them cool on a wire rack. MAKES ABOUT 2 DOZEN COOKIES

REDUCED-SUGAR CHOCOLATE–COCONUT-OATMEAL COOKIES

Make the Chocolate–Coconut-Oatmeal Cookies (above) as described, but reduce the brown sugar to ½ cup (115 g) and add ⅛ teaspoon of stevia.

Pecan-Coconut Bars

BOTTOM LAYER:

Coconut oil or coconut oil–based nonstick cooking spray, to coat the baking pan

1 cup (225 g) firmly packed dark brown sugar

1 cup (2 sticks/225 g) salted butter, softened

2 large eggs

1 teaspoon vanilla extract

2 cups (250 g) flour, plus extra flour to dust your hands

¼ teaspoon salt

TOP LAYER:

½ cup (115 g) sucanat or firmly packed dark brown sugar

2 tablespoons (15 g) flour

¼ cup (½ stick/55 or 60 ml) salted butter or coconut oil, softened

½ cup (56 g) pecans

½ cup (42 g) flaked coconut

PREHEAT THE OVEN TO 350°F (180°C). Coat a 13 x 9 x 2-inch (33 x 23 x 5-cm) baking pan with a thin layer of coconut oil or nonstick cooking spray. For the bottom layer, in a medium bowl, mix together the brown sugar, butter, eggs, and vanilla. Stir in the flour and salt. With your hands, press the batter into the prepared pan. To prevent dough from sticking to your hands, keep them dry by dusting them in flour. Set aside.

For the top layer, in a small bowl, mix together brown sugar, flour, butter, pecans, and flaked coconut, and spread evenly over the bottom layer. Bake for 35 to 40 minutes, or until a knife inserted in the center comes out clean. Cool, and then cut into bars.   MAKES 12 BARS

REDUCED-SUGAR PECAN-COCONUT BARS

Make the bottom layer of the Pecan-Coconut Bars (page 183) as directed, except reduce the brown sugar to ½ cup (115 g) and the butter to ¾ cup (167 g). Make the top layer as directed, but reduce the brown sugar to ¼ cup (60 g).

Chocolate-Coconut Bars ⊛

Coconut oil or coconut oil–based nonstick cooking spray,
    to coat the baking pan
1 cup (225 g) firmly packed dark brown sugar
1 cup (2 sticks/225 g) butter, softened
2 large eggs
1 teaspoon vanilla extract
2 cups (250 g) flour, plus more for dusting your hands
¼ teaspoon salt
½ cup (55 g) chopped almonds, toasted
⅔ cup (166 g) milk chocolate chips
1 cup (85 g) flaked coconut, toasted

PREHEAT THE OVEN TO 350°F (180°C). Coat a 13 x 9 x 2-inch (33 x 23 x 5-cm) baking pan with a thin layer of coconut oil or nonstick cooking spray. In a medium bowl, mix together the brown sugar, butter, eggs, and vanilla. Stir in the flour and salt; add the toasted almonds. With your hands, press the batter into the prepared pan. To prevent dough from sticking to your hands, keep them dry by dusting them in flour. Bake for 25 to 30 minutes, or until very light brown. Remove from the oven. Sprinkle the chocolate chips over the hot crust. Let stand until the chips soften; then spread the chocolate evenly over the crust. Sprinkle the top with toasted coconut.

MAKES 16 BARS

REDUCED-SUGAR CHOCOLATE-COCONUT BARS
Make the Chocolate-Coconut Bars (page 184) as directed, but reduce the brown sugar to ½ cup (115 g) and add ⅛ teaspoon of stevia. Sprinkle toasted coconut on top as directed.

Coconut Sugar Cookies

> Coconut oil–based nonstick cooking spray or coconut oil,
>   to coat the baking sheet
> 3 cups (375 g) flour, plus more to dust the work surface
> 1½ teaspoons baking powder
> 1 teaspoon salt
> 1¼ cups (300 ml) coconut oil, melted
> 1½ cups (300 g) sugar
> 1½ teaspoons almond extract
> 3 large eggs
> 1½ cups (128 g) grated coconut

PREHEAT THE OVEN TO 375°F (190°C). Lightly coat a baking sheet with coconut oil or nonstick cooking spray. In a medium bowl, mix the flour, baking powder, and salt; set aside. In a separate bowl, combine the coconut oil, sugar, and almond extract. Add the eggs, one at a time, beating well after each addition. Add the coconut and slowly mix the wet ingredients into the dry ingredients until just blended. If your kitchen is very hot, wrap the dough in wax paper and chill for about 1 hour so it will roll more easily. Roll a quarter of the dough at a time on a lightly floured board to a thickness of about ¼ inch (6 mm). Use a cookie cutter or the top of a drinking glass to cut out the cookies. Using a pancake turner, transfer the cookie dough to the prepared baking sheet, spacing the cookies 2 inches (5 cm) apart. Bake for 12 to 15 minutes, until pale tan. Transfer the cookies to wire racks to cool. MAKES ABOUT 3 DOZEN COOKIES

REDUCED-SUGAR COCONUT SUGAR COOKIES
Make the Coconut Sugar Cookies (page 185) as directed, but reduce the sugar to ¾ cup (150 g) and add ⅛ teaspoon of stevia. MAKES ABOUT 3 DOZEN COOKIES

Almond-Coconut Cookies

> 2 large eggs, separated
> 1 cup (2 sticks/225 g) salted butter, softened
> 1½ cups (340 g) sucanat or firmly packed dark brown sugar
> ½ teaspoon almond extract
> 2½ cups (312 g) flour
> ¾ cup (82 g) chopped almonds
> 1 teaspoon baking powder
> 2 teaspoons cream of tartar
> ¼ teaspoon salt
> Shredded or flaked coconut

PREHEAT THE OVEN TO 350°F (180°C). In a medium bowl, mix together the egg yolks with the butter, sucanat, and almond extract; set aside. In a separate bowl, mix together the flour, almonds, baking powder, cream of tartar, and salt. Stir together the wet ingredients and dry ingredients. Roll the dough into 1½-inch (3.5-cm) balls and dip them into the egg whites, then into the coconut. Place them on an ungreased baking sheet. Bake for 12 to 15 minutes, or until the coconut is lightly browned. Remove from the baking sheet immediately and cool on a wire rack.   MAKES ABOUT 3 DOZEN COOKIES

REDUCED-SUGAR ALMOND-COCONUT COOKIES
Make the Almond Coconut Cookies (page 186) according to the directions, but reduce the sucanat to ¾ cup (170 g) and add ⅛ teaspoon of stevia. MAKES ABOUT 3 DOZEN COOKIES

Apricot-Coconut Bars ⚙

    Coconut oil or coconut oil–based nonstick cooking spray,
       to coat the baking pan

    1 cup (225 g) firmly packed dark brown sugar

    1 cup (2 sticks/224 g) salted butter or coconut oil, melted

    2 large eggs

    1 teaspoon vanilla extract

    2 cups (250 g) flour, plus more for dusting your hands

    ¼ teaspoon salt

    1 cup (320 g) apricot jam or preserves

    ½ cup (60 g) chopped walnuts

    ½ cup (42 g) flaked coconut

PREHEAT THE OVEN TO 350°F (180°C). Coat a 13 x 9 x 2-inch (33 x 23 x 5-cm) baking pan with a thin layer of coconut oil or nonstick cooking spray. In a medium bowl, mix together the brown sugar, butter, eggs, and vanilla. Stir in the flour and salt. With your hands, press the dough into the prepared baking pan. To prevent the dough from sticking to your hands, keep them dry by dusting them in flour. Spread an even layer of apricot jam over the batter. Cover the jam with the walnuts and coconut. Bake for 35 to 40 minutes, or until a knife inserted in the center comes out clean. Cool and cut into bars.   MAKES 16 BARS

REDUCED-SUGAR APRICOT-COCONUT BARS

Make the Apricot-Coconut Bars (above) according to recipe, but reduce the brown sugar to ½ cup (115 g) and add ⅛ teaspoon of stevia. Use "low sugar" apricot preserves. Smucker's makes an apricot preserve with 50 percent less sugar than what is usually used.

Haystacks

These cookies look much like miniature stacks of hay and taste very similar to coconut macaroons.

> Coconut oil or coconut oil–based nonstick cooking spray,
>> to coat the baking sheet
> ¼ cup (½ stick/56 g) salted butter or coconut oil, melted
> 1 cup (200 g) sugar
> 4 large eggs
> ½ teaspoon vanilla extract
> ¼ teaspoon almond extract
> ¼ cup (31 g) flour
> 4 cups (340 g) grated or flaked coconut

PREHEAT THE OVEN TO 375°F (190°C). Coat a baking sheet with a thin layer of coconut oil or nonstick cooking spray. In a medium bowl, mix together the butter, sugar, eggs, vanilla, and almond extract. Stir in the flour and coconut. Drop the dough in spoon-size mounds about 1 inch (2.5 cm) apart onto the prepared baking sheet. Bake for 18 to 20 minutes, or until golden brown. Remove from the baking sheet immediately and cool on a wire rack.

MAKES ABOUT 30 HAYSTACKS

CHOCOLATE HAYSTACKS

Make the Haystacks (above) according to the directions, but add ½ cup (88 g) of milk chocolate chips to the batter.

BUTTERSCOTCH HAYSTACKS

Make the Haystacks (above) according to the directions, but add ½ cup (133 g) of butterscotch chips to the batter.

REDUCED-SUGAR HAYSTACKS

Make the Haystacks (above) according to the directions, but reduce the sugar to ½ cup (100 g) and add ⅛ teaspoon of stevia.

Coconut Sesame Balls ✿

> ¼ cup (36 g) sesame seeds
> ¼ cup (38 g) sunflower seeds
> ¾ cup (64 g) shredded coconut
> 3 tablespoons (48 g) peanut butter (see Note)
> 2 tablespoons (27 g) rice syrup (see Note)

PREHEAT THE OVEN TO 350°F (180°C). Put the sesame seeds and sunflower seeds on a rimmed baking sheet. Put the coconut on a second rimmed baking sheet. Bake the seeds and coconut for about 8 to 12 minutes, or until lightly toasted. Coconut cooks more quickly and will need to be taken out of the oven first. In a medium bowl, blend the peanut butter and rice syrup. Add the toasted sesame seeds, sunflower seeds, and coconut, and mix together. Spoon the mixture into bite-size balls and place on wax paper. Chill them in the refrigerator to harden.   **MAKES ABOUT 16 BALLS**

Note

You may substitute tahini or almond butter for the peanut butter if you desire.

You may substitute 1 tablespoon (20 g) honey for the rice syrup in this recipe, but the balls will be softer and a little more difficult to shape.

Chocolate Crisps ✿

This is one of those treats that should be reserved for those with a great deal of willpower. They're so unbelievably good that you can't eat just one.

> 1 cup (110 g) chopped almonds
> 1 cup (85 g) flaked coconut
> 2 cups (350 g) milk chocolate chips

PREHEAT THE OVEN TO 350°F (180°C). Place the almonds on a rimmed baking sheet. Place the coconut on a second rimmed baking sheet. Toast the almonds and coconut in the oven for about 8 to 10 minutes. (Use 2 separate baking sheets because the coconut toasts more quickly.) In a medium saucepan, melt the chocolate chips over low heat, stirring frequently. Don't overcook; heat just until slightly melted. When the chocolate is soft, remove it from the heat and stir in the toasted almonds and coconut. Drop by the tablespoon onto wax paper and cool. If your kitchen is too warm, you may need to put them in the refrigerator to set. Store in a cool place or in the refrigerator.   MAKES ABOUT 15 CRISPS

CHOCOLATE CRISPIES
Make the Chocolate Crisps (page 189) as directed, but replace the almonds with 1 cup (28 g) of crisp rice cereal.

PEANUT BUTTER CRISPIES
Make the Chocolate Crisps (page 189) as directed, with the crisp rice cereal, and add ½ cup (130 g) of peanut butter.

ROCKY ROAD CRISPS
Make the Chocolate Crisps (page 189) as directed, but substitute 1 cup (112 g) of pecans for the almonds and add 1 cup (50 g) of miniature marshmallows.

Granola Bars

Coconut oil to coat the baking pan
Flour for dusting the baking pan
3½ cups (280 g) old-fashioned oats
1 cup (85 g) flaked coconut
1 cup (145 g) raisins
1 cup (about 120 g) chopped nuts
⅔ cup (150 g) salted butter, softened
½ cup (115 g) sucanat or firmly packed dark brown sugar
⅓ cup (115 g) corn syrup or honey
½ teaspoon salt
1 large egg, beaten
½ teaspoon vanilla extract

PREHEAT THE OVEN TO 325°F (170°C). Coat a 13 x 9 x 2-inch (33 x 23 x 5-cm) baking pan with a thin layer of coconut oil and dust with flour. In a large bowl, mix together the oats, coconut, raisins, nuts, butter, sucanat, corn syrup, and salt. In a separate bowl, combine the egg and vanilla, then stir it into the coconut mix. Press the granola firmly into the prepared baking pan. Bake for 40 minutes. Remove from the oven and let cool completely. Cut into bars. MAKES 16 BARS

REDUCED-SUGAR GRANOLA BARS

Make the Granola Bars (page 190) as directed, but delete the sucanat and corn syrup and add ½ cup (108 g) of rice syrup and ⅛ teaspoon of stevia.

Chocolate Granola Bars ⚙

Coconut oil, to coat the baking pan

Flour for dusting the baking pan

1 cup (110 g) chopped almonds

⅔ cup (150 g) salted butter, softened

3½ cups (280 g) old-fashioned oats

1 cup (85 g) flaked coconut

½ cup (88 g) semisweet chocolate chips

½ cup (115 g) sucanat or firmly packed dark brown sugar

⅓ cup (115 g) corn syrup or honey

½ teaspoon salt

1 large egg, beaten

½ teaspoon vanilla extract

PREHEAT THE OVEN TO 350°F (180°C). Coat a 13 x 9 x 2-inch (33 x 23 x 5-cm) baking pan with a thin layer of coconut oil and dust with flour. Place the almonds on a rimmed baking sheet and toast in the oven for 10 minutes. Remove the almonds from the oven and reduce the oven temperature to 325°F (170°C). In a medium bowl, mix together the toasted almonds, butter, oats, coconut, chocolate chips, sucanat, corn syrup, and salt. In a small bowl, combine the egg and vanilla; stir the egg mixture into the nut mixture. Press the granola firmly into the prepared baking pan. Bake for 40 minutes. Remove from the oven and let cool completely. Cut into bars.

MAKES 16 BARS

Coconut Butter Cookies

> 3 cups (375 g) flour
>
> 1½ cups (128 g) grated coconut
>
> 1½ teaspoons baking powder
>
> 1 teaspoon salt
>
> 1 cup (2 sticks/225 g) unsalted butter, softened
>
> 1½ cups (300 g) sugar
>
> 2 teaspoons vanilla extract
>
> 3 large eggs

PREHEAT THE OVEN TO 375°F (190°C). In a large bowl, mix the flour, coconut, baking powder, and salt; set aside. In another bowl, blend the butter, sugar, vanilla, and eggs. Mix together the wet ingredients and the dry ingredients. Form the dough into balls 1½ inches (4 cm) in diameter. Place on an ungreased baking sheet 2 inches (5 cm) apart. Bake for 12 to 15 minutes, until pale tan. Transfer to wire racks to cool.

MAKES ABOUT 3 DOZEN COOKIES

PIES

Pastry

Coconut Oil Pastry

Using coconut oil to make piecrust produces excellent results. The following recipes are for a single-crust and a double-crust 8-, 9-, or 10-inch (20-, 23-, or 25-cm) pie. These recipes work equally well with either whole-wheat or white flour. The only difference is that whole-wheat crusts often need 1 to 2 tablespoons (15 to 30 ml) more water than white-flour crusts. The secret to making good piecrusts using coconut oil is to chill the oil before cutting it into the flour. The kitchen should be 72°F (22°C) or cooler for best results. If you have a food processor, cutting the oil into the flour is quick and simple.

Single Crust

1¼ cups (156 g) flour, plus more for the work surface and rolling pin

½ teaspoon salt

⅓ cup (80 ml) chilled coconut oil

4 to 5 tablespoons (60 to 75 ml) ice water, or 5 to 6 tablespoons
(75 to 90 ml) if using whole-wheat flour

Double Crust

2 cups (250 g) flour, plus more for the work surface and rolling pin

1 teaspoon salt

⅔ cup (145 g) chilled coconut oil

5 to 7 tablespoons (75 to 105 ml) ice water, or 7 to 8 tablespoons
(105 to 120 ml) if using whole-wheat flour

IN A LARGE BOWL, mix together the flour and salt. In the bowl of a food processor, combine the flour mixture and the hardened coconut oil. Process until the pieces are between the size of small peas and coarse cornmeal. If you don't have a food processor, you can mix it by hand with a pastry blender or a fork and knife. Gradually add ice water, a tablespoon at a time, until the pastry is moistened and begins to stick together and not to the container.

Put a strip of wax paper on a flat surface. Tape the edges of the paper down so it doesn't move. Lightly flour the surface of the wax paper. Gather the pastry into a ball; flatten it out on the wax paper. Lightly flour a rolling pin and flatten the pastry until about ⅛ inch (3 mm) thick. (For a two-crust pie, divide the pastry into halves and shape each individually.) Add more flour to the rolling pin as needed to prevent the pastry from sticking.

Lift the wax paper from the flat surface with one hand underneath the paper and one on the pastry, and gently turn it upside down into the pie plate (or fold half of the pastry over the pin and ease it into the pan). Remove the wax paper and shape the crust into the pie plate, pressing firmly against the bottom and sides. Seal any cracks or holes by pressing dampened scraps of pastry on top. Trim the overhanging edge of pastry and flute as desired. Fill and bake as directed in the recipe.

BAKED SINGLE-CRUST PIE SHELL

Prick the bottom and side thoroughly with a fork to avoid shrinkage and distortion of the shell during baking. Bake at 450°F (230°C) for 10 to 12 minutes, until lightly browned.

DOUBLE-CRUST PIE

Leave a 1-inch (2.5 cm) trim of top pastry beyond the edge of the pie plate. Fold and roll the rim of the top pastry under the edge of the bottom pastry, then press together to seal. The edge can be fluted in any manner you wish for an attractive finish. Cut several slits in the top crust to allow steam to escape. Bake as directed in the recipe.

TART PASTRY SHELLS

Tarts are basically miniature pies. Each pie is an individual serving. Prepare the pastry as you would for a full-size pie. If you want to make 4 double-crust tart shells, use the Double-Crust recipe. Divide the pastry into 8 balls. Roll them out into 5- to 6-inch (13 to 15 cm) circles and place the bottom crust into 4 tart pans or custard cups. Fill the tarts with filling and cover with a top crust. Bake as directed in the recipe. You can use tart shells to make any of the pie recipes that follow.

Coconut Pastry Shell

This pastry shell contains grated coconut.

> 1 cup (125 g) flour
> ½ cup (42 g) grated coconut
> ¼ teaspoon salt
> ½ cup (109 g) chilled coconut oil
> 3 to 4 (45 to 60 ml) tablespoons ice water

IN A MEDIUM BOWL, mix the flour, coconut, and salt together. Follow the Coconut Oil Pastry recipe (page 193), using the flour/coconut mixture.

MAKES 1 SINGLE CRUST

Toppings

Meringue

> 3 large egg whites
> ½ teaspoon vanilla extract
> ¼ teaspoon cream of tartar
> ¼ cup (50 g) sugar

PREHEAT THE OVEN TO 350°F (180°C). In the bowl of a standing mixer, beat the egg whites, vanilla, and cream of tartar at high speed for about 4 minutes, until soft peaks form. Gradually add the sugar, beating until stiff and the sugar is dissolved. Spread the meringue over the hot pie filling, spreading it all the way to the edge of the pastry (this helps prevent the meringue from shrinking). Bake for 12 to 15 minutes, or until the meringue is golden brown. Cool.   MAKES ABOUT 1½ CUPS

REDUCED-SUGAR MERINGUE

Make the Meringue (page 195) as directed, but reduce the sugar to 2 tablespoons (26 g) and add a dash of powdered stevia extract. Use just a tiny bit and gradually add more if you want the meringue to be sweeter; a little can go a long way and too much will give the meringue a bitter aftertaste.

Coconut Whipped Cream ✿

This recipe uses a mixture of heavy whipping cream and coconut cream.

> ½ cup plus 2 tablespoons (150 ml) heavy cream
> ½ teaspoon imitation coconut extract or 1 teaspoon vanilla extract
> 3 tablespoons (11 g) confectioners' sugar
> ½ cup (120 ml) coconut cream (see Note)

IN A MEDIUM-SIZE BOWL, combine the heavy cream and coconut extract. Using an electric mixer, whip the cream at high speed until soft peaks form. Add the sugar and beat until stiff peaks form. Whip in the coconut cream. This may cause it to lose some of its volume, depending on the thickness of the coconut cream, but that's okay. Chill and serve cold.

MAKES ABOUT 1½ CUPS (280 G)

Note

If you don't have coconut cream, you can use coconut milk. Use the creamiest portion of the milk. The thickness of the coconut cream you use will determine the thickness of the whipped cream you end up with. The cream in many brands of coconut milk naturally separates out and rises to the top. When you open a can of coconut milk, you can scoop out the cream. Be careful not to shake the can before opening. Refrigerating coconut milk for several days before opening causes more of the cream to separate and rise to the top.

ALMOND WHIPPED CREAM

Prepare the Coconut Whipped Cream (page 196) as directed, but replace the coconut extract with ½ teaspoon of almond extract.

PEPPERMINT WHIPPED CREAM

Prepare the Coconut Whipped Cream (page 196) as directed, but replace the coconut extract with ½ teaspoon of peppermint extract.

MAPLE WHIPPED CREAM

Prepare the Coconut Whipped Cream (page 196) as directed, but replace the coconut extract with ¼ teaspoon of maple flavoring.

CHOCOLATE WHIPPED CREAM

Prepare the Coconut Whipped Cream (page 196) as directed, but add 3 tablespoons (16 g) of cocoa powder, increase the confectioners' sugar to 6 tablespoons (22 g), and use ½ teaspoon of vanilla extract and ½ teaspoon of imitation coconut extract.

REDUCED-SUGAR COCONUT WHIPPED CREAM

Prepare the Coconut Whipped Cream (page 196) as directed, but reduce the confectioners' sugar to 1 tablespoon (4 g) and add a pinch or two of powdered stevia extract. Use just a tiny bit and gradually add more if you want it sweeter; a little can go a long way and too much will give the whipped cream a bitter aftertaste.

Pies

Super-Delicious Coconut Pie ✿

This is a delicious and easy-to-make pie.

> 3 large eggs, beaten
> 2 tablespoons (15 g) flour
> 1½ cups (300 g) sugar
> ½ cup (1 stick/112 g) unsalted butter, melted
> 4 teaspoons freshly squeezed lemon juice
> 1 teaspoon vanilla extract
> 1⅓ cups (113 g) grated coconut
> Dash of salt
> 1 9-inch (23-cm) unbaked pastry shell
> Coconut Whipped Cream (page 196)

PREHEAT THE OVEN TO 350°F (180°C). In a large bowl, combine the eggs, flour, sugar, butter, lemon juice, vanilla, coconut, and salt and mix well. Pour into the unbaked pastry shell and bake for 40 to 45 minutes, until the top forms a golden crust and a knife inserted in the center comes out clean. Cool and top with Coconut Whipped Cream (page 196).   SERVES 8

REDUCED-SUGAR SUPER-DELICIOUS COCONUT PIE

Make the Super-Delicious Coconut Pie (above) as directed, but reduce the sugar to ¾ cup (150 g), add up to ⅛ teaspoon of stevia, and reduce the lemon juice to 3 teaspoons. This may be served with or without whipped cream; it's good either way.

Frozen Coconut Pie ✿

> ½ cup (100 g) sugar
> ¾ cup (175 ml) coconut milk
> 1¼ cups (106 g) flaked coconut
> ½ teaspoon almond extract
> 1½ cups (90 g) Coconut Whipped Cream (page 196)
> 1 9-inch (23-cm) baked pastry shell

IN A MEDIUM BOWL, combine the sugar, coconut milk, coconut, and almond extract. Let the mixture sit for about 5 minutes to allow the sugar to dissolve. Fold in the Coconut Whipped Cream. Pour into the baked pastry shell and freeze for at least 4 hours. Thaw for 15 minutes before serving.   SERVES 8

FROZEN CHOCOLATE-COCONUT PIE

Make the Frozen Coconut Pie (page 198) as directed, but reduce the coconut milk to ½ cup (120 ml) and the flaked coconut to 1 cup (85 g). Replace the Coconut Whipped Cream with 2½ cups (1 recipe) (250 g) of Chocolate Whipped Cream (page 197).

Vanilla Cream Pie

   ¾ cup (150 g) sugar

   3 tablespoons (24 g) cornstarch

   ¼ teaspoon salt

   1 can (14 ounces/400 ml) coconut milk

   3 large egg yolks, slightly beaten (Note: Use the 3 egg whites for the Meringue.)

   2 tablespoons (¼ stick/28 g) unsalted butter

   1 tablespoon (15 ml) vanilla extract

   1 9-inch (23-cm) baked pastry shell

   Meringue (page 195)

PREHEAT THE OVEN TO 350°F (180°C). In a medium saucepan, combine the sugar, cornstarch, and salt; stir in the coconut milk. Cook and stir over medium heat until bubbly; cook and stir for 2 minutes more. Remove from the heat. Slowly stir at least ½ cup (120 ml) of the hot mixture into the egg yolks and immediately return the egg yolk mixture to the hot mixture; cook for 4 minutes over medium heat, stirring constantly. Remove from the heat. Add the butter and vanilla. Pour the mixture into the cooled baked pastry shell. Spread the meringue on top of the pie and bake for 12 to 15 minutes, until the meringue is a golden brown. Cool and store in the refrigerator. Serve chilled.   SERVES 8

CHOCOLATE CREAM PIE

Prepare the Vanilla Cream Pie (page 199), increasing the sugar to 1 cup (200 g). Add 2 1-ounce (29-g) squares of unsweetened chocolate with the coconut milk. Top with Meringue (page 196) and bake as directed.

BANANA CREAM PIE

Slice 3 bananas and put into a cooled baked 9-inch (23-cm) pastry shell. Add the Vanilla Cream Pie filling (above) or Chocolate Cream Pie filling (above). Top with Meringue (page 196) and bake as directed.

COCONUT CREAM PIE

Add 1 cup (85 g) of grated coconut to the Vanilla Cream Pie filling (page 199). Cover with Meringue (page 196) and sprinkle the top with ⅓ cup (28 g) of shredded or flaked coconut. Bake as directed.

PEPPERMINT CREAM PIE

Add 1 teaspoon of peppermint extract to the Vanilla Cream Pie filling (page 199). Top with Meringue (page 196) or Peppermint Whipped Cream (page 197). Serve with crushed peppermint candy sprinkled on top.

CARAMEL CREAM PIE

Prepare the Vanilla Cream Pie (page 199), replacing the granulated sugar with sucanat.

REDUCED-SUGAR CREAM PIES

Make the pie as directed, but reduce the sugar to ⅓ cup (66 g) and add ⅛ teaspoon of stevia. For reduced-sugar Chocolate Cream Pie, use ¾ cup sugar (150 g) and enough stevia to suit your taste.

Lemon Chiffon Pie

1 envelope (4-ounce/7-g) unflavored gelatin

1 cup (200 g) sugar

½ teaspoon salt

4 large egg yolks

⅓ cup (80 ml) freshly squeezed lemon juice

⅓ cup (80 ml) water

⅔ cup (160 ml) coconut milk

½ teaspoon grated lemon peel

4 large egg whites

⅛ teaspoon cream of tartar

1 9-inch (23-cm) baked pastry shell, cooled

IN A MEDIUM SAUCEPAN, combine the gelatin, ½ cup (100 g) of the sugar, and the salt. In another bowl, mix together the egg yolks, lemon juice, water, and coconut milk. Stir the egg yolk mixture into the gelatin mixture. Cook over medium heat, stirring constantly, until the mixture comes to a boil and the gelatin dissolves. Remove from the heat and stir in the lemon peel. Chill in the refrigerator, stirring occasionally, for about 45 minutes, until partially set but still pourable. In the bowl of a standing mixer, combine the egg whites and cream of tartar. Beat the egg whites at high speed until soft peaks form. Gradually add the remaining ½ cup (100 g) of sugar, beating until stiff peaks form. Fold in the partially set gelatin mixture. Pour the entire mixture into the cooled baked pastry shell. Chill until firm, about 3 to 5 hours.   SERVES 8

Strawberry Chiffon Pie ✿

2 cups (340 g) sliced fresh strawberries

½ cup (100 g) sugar

⅓ cup (80 ml) water

1 envelope (4-ounce/7-g) unflavored gelatin

⅔ cup (160 ml) coconut milk

1 tablespoon freshly squeezed lemon juice

Dash of salt

2 large egg whites

⅛ teaspoon cream of tartar

1 9-inch (23-cm) baked pastry shell, cooled

IN A MEDIUM BOWL, crush the strawberries; add ¼ cup (50 g) of the sugar; let stand for 30 minutes. In the meantime, in a small saucepan, bring the water to a boil over medium heat, remove from the heat, and let sit for

1 minute. Stir in the gelatin and allow to cool, about 5 minutes. Add the gelatin, coconut milk, lemon juice, and salt to the strawberry mix. Chill in the refrigerator, stirring occasionally, for about 45 minutes, until partially set but still pourable. In the bowl of a standing mixer, add the egg whites and cream of tartar. Beat the egg whites at high speed until soft peaks form; gradually add the remaining ¼ cup (50 g) of sugar, beating until stiff peaks form. Fold the egg whites into the strawberry mixture. Fill the cooled baked pastry shell with the strawberry mixture. Chill until firm, 3 to 5 hours.
SERVES 8

REDUCED-SUGAR STRAWBERRY CHIFFON PIE
Make the Strawberry Chiffon Pie (page 201) as directed, but increase the strawberries to 3 cups (510 g), reduce the lemon juice to 2 teaspoons, reduce the sugar in the gelatin mixture to 1 tablespoon (13 g), add ⅛ teaspoon of stevia, and reduce the sugar in the egg whites to 2 tablespoons (26 g). You may adjust the amount of sugar and stevia to suit your taste.

Chocolate Chiffon Pie

> 1 envelope (4-ounce/7-g) unflavored gelatin
> ¼ cup (60 ml) cold water
> 3 large egg yolks
> ¼ teaspoon salt
> 1 teaspoon vanilla extract
> ¾ cup (150 g) sugar
> 2 1-ounce (29 g) squares unsweetened chocolate
> ½ cup (120 ml) coconut milk
> 3 large egg whites
> ⅛ teaspoon cream of tartar
> 1 9-inch (23-cm) baked pastry shell, cooled
> Coconut Whipped Cream (page 196), for topping

IN A SMALL BOWL, soften the gelatin in the cold water. In the bowl of a standing mixer, beat together the egg yolks at high speed, then gradually beat in the salt, vanilla, and ½ cup (100 g) of the sugar. In a medium saucepan, combine the chocolate and coconut milk; stir over low heat until melted.

Add the softened gelatin and stir to dissolve. Add the egg yolk mixture to the chocolate mixture and combine; remove from the heat. Chill in the refrigerator, stirring occasionally, for about 45 minutes, until the mixture is partially set but still pourable. In a separate bowl of a standing mixer, combine the egg whites and cream of tartar. Beat the egg whites at high speed until soft peaks form. Gradually add the remaining ¼ cup (50 g) of sugar, beating until stiff peaks form. Add the egg whites to the chilled chocolate mixture; fold in just until blended. Fill the baked pie shell. Chill until firm, 3 to 5 hours. Top with whipped cream.   SERVES 8

Black-Bottom–Custard Pie

BOTTOM LAYER:

 1 can (14 ounces/400 ml) coconut milk
 4 large egg yolks, beaten
 ½ cup (100 g) sugar
 2 tablespoons (16 g) cornstarch
 1 teaspoon vanilla extract
 1 6-ounce package (1 cup/175 g) semisweet chocolate chips
 1 9-inch (23-cm) baked pastry shell

TOP LAYER:

 1 envelope (4-ounce/7-g) unflavored gelatin
 ¼ cup (60 ml) water
 ½ teaspoon almond extract
 4 large egg whites
 ½ cup (100 g) sugar
 Sliced almonds, toasted

FOR THE BOTTOM LAYER, in a medium saucepan, mix the coconut milk and egg yolks together. Stir in the sugar and cornstarch. Cook and stir over medium heat for about 5 minutes, until the custard thickens. Remove from the heat and add the vanilla. Put 1 cup (235 ml) of the hot custard in a separate bowl, along with the chocolate chips; stir until melted (you will have some custard left over to be used below). Pour the mixture into the baked pastry shell and chill.

Meanwhile, for the top layer, in a small bowl, soften the gelatin by combining it with the water and the remaining hot custard. Stir until dissolved. Mix in the almond extract. Chill for about 30 minutes, until slightly thickened. In a medium bowl, beat the egg whites at high speed until soft peaks form; gradually add the sugar; beat again until stiff peaks form. Fold the egg white mixture into the chilled custard-gelatin mixture. Remove the half-filled pie from the refrigerator and pour the mixture on top of the chocolate layer. Sprinkle the top with lightly toasted sliced almonds. Chill for 3 to 4 hours, until set.   SERVES 8

Coconut Custard Pie

4 large eggs, slightly beaten
2 tablespoons (15 g) flour
½ cup (100 g) sugar
¼ teaspoon salt
1 tablespoon (15 ml) vanilla extract
1 can (14 ounces/400 ml) coconut milk
1 9-inch (23-cm) unbaked pastry shell
1 cup (85 g) flaked coconut

PREHEAT THE OVEN TO 350°F (180°C). In a large bowl, blend together the eggs, flour, sugar, salt, and vanilla. Stir in the coconut milk. Pour into the unbaked pastry shell. Sprinkle the top with flaked coconut. Bake for about 60 minutes, or until a knife inserted in the center comes out clean. Cool on a rack, then chill.   SERVES 8

REDUCED-SUGAR COCONUT CUSTARD PIE

Make the Coconut Custard Pie (above) as directed, but reduce the sugar to ¼ cup (50 g) and add a dash or two of stevia or enough to suit your taste.

Lemon Meringue Pie ⚙

> 1 can (14 ounces/400 ml) coconut milk
> 1½ cups (300 g) sugar
> ⅓ cup plus 1 tablespoon (50 g) cornstarch
> 3 large egg yolks, slightly beaten
> 3 tablespoons (42 g) salted butter
> ½ teaspoon grated lemon peel
> ½ cup (120 ml) freshly squeezed lemon juice
> 1 9-inch (23-cm) baked pastry shell
> Meringue (page 196)

PREHEAT THE OVEN TO 400°F (200°C). In a medium saucepan, mix together the coconut milk, sugar, and cornstarch. Cook over medium heat, stirring constantly, until the mixture thickens and begins to boil. Cook and stir for 1 minute. Remove from the heat. Gradually stir at least half of the hot mixture into the egg yolks and then stir the egg yolks into the rest of the hot mixture in the saucepan. Return to medium heat and cook for 1 minute, stirring constantly. Remove from the heat; stir in the butter, lemon peel, and lemon juice. Pour the mixture into the baked pie shell. Spoon the meringue on top of the hot pie filling; spread the meringue over the filling, carefully sealing the meringue to the edge of the crust to prevent shrinking. Bake for 10 minutes, or until light brown. Cool on a wire rack and then place in the refrigerator. Serve chilled.   SERVES 8

Orange Meringue Pie

> 1 can (14 ounces/400 ml) coconut milk
> 1½ cups (300 g) sugar
> ⅓ cup plus 1 tablespoon (50 g) cornstarch
> 3 large egg yolks, slightly beaten
> 3 tablespoons (42 g) unsalted butter
> 1 teaspoon grated orange peel
> ¼ cup (60 ml) freshly squeezed orange juice
> ¼ cup (60 ml) freshly squeezed lemon juice

1 9-inch (23-cm) baked pastry shell
Meringue (page 196)

PREHEAT THE OVEN TO 400°F (200°C). In a medium saucepan, mix together the coconut milk, sugar, and cornstarch. Cook over medium heat, stirring constantly, until the mixture thickens and begins to boil. Cook and stir for 1 minute. Remove from the heat. Gradually stir at least half of the hot mixture into the egg yolks and then stir the egg yolks into the rest of the hot mixture in the saucepan. Return to medium heat and cook for 1 minute, stirring constantly. Remove from the heat; stir in the butter, orange peel, orange juice, and lemon juice. Pour the mixture into the baked pie shell. Spoon the meringue on top of the hot pie filling; spread the meringue over the filling, carefully sealing the meringue to the edge of the crust to prevent shrinking. Bake for 10 minutes, or until light brown. Cool on a wire rack and then place in the refrigerator. Serve chilled.   SERVES 8

Coconut-Lime Pie

4 large egg yolks
½ cup (100 g) sugar
2 teaspoons salt
⅓ cup (80 ml) freshly squeezed lime juice (2 to 3 limes)
1 cup (60 g) Coconut Whipped Cream (page 196), plus more for
     topping
1 tablespoon (6 g) grated lime peel
1 9-inch (23-cm) baked pastry shell

IN A SMALL BOWL, beat together the egg yolks and transfer them to a medium saucepan. Add the sugar, salt, and lime juice. Cook over medium heat, stirring constantly, for about 5 minutes, until the mixture thickens. Remove from the heat and chill in the refrigerator. Fold in the Coconut Whipped Cream and lime peel. Spoon into the baked pastry shell; refrigerate for at least 4 hours. Top with Coconut Whipped Cream.   SERVES 8

Pumpkin Pie

1 can (15 to 16 ounces/459 to 490 g) pumpkin

¾ cup (150 g) sugar

¾ teaspoon salt

1 teaspoon ground cinnamon

½ teaspoon ground ginger

¼ teaspoon ground nutmeg

¼ teaspoon ground cloves

3 large eggs, slightly beaten

1 cup (235 ml) coconut milk

1 9-inch (23-cm) unbaked pastry shell

Coconut Whipped Cream (page 196), for topping

PREHEAT THE OVEN TO 400°F (200°C). In a medium bowl, mix together the pumpkin, sugar, salt, cinnamon, ginger, nutmeg, cloves, eggs, and coconut milk; pour the mixture into the pastry shell. The Coconut Pastry Shell (page 195) works well for this pie. Bake for about 50 minutes, or until a knife inserted in the center comes out clean. Cool. Just before serving, top with Coconut Whipped Cream (page 196).   SERVES 8

SWEET POTATO PIE

Prepare the Pumpkin Pie (above) as directed, but substitute 1½ cups (382.5 g) of cooked mashed sweet potatoes for the pumpkin.

REDUCED-SUGAR PUMPKIN PIE

Make the Pumpkin Pie (above) as directed, but reduce the sugar to ½ cup (100 g), add ⅛ teaspoon of stevia, and add 1 tablespoon (8 g) of flour.

Coconut-Pecan Pie ✿

4 large eggs, beaten

1 cup (200 g) sugar

½ cup (1 stick/120 ml) salted butter, melted

4 teaspoons freshly squeezed lemon juice

1 teaspoon vanilla extract

1 cup (85 g) grated coconut

1 9-inch (23-cm) unbaked pastry shell
⅔ cup (70 g) pecan halves

PREHEAT THE OVEN TO 350°F (180°C). In a large bowl, beat together the eggs, sugar, butter, lemon juice, and vanilla until well blended; stir in the coconut. Pour into the unbaked pie shell. Carefully layer the pecan halves on top of the pie filling. Bake for 40 minutes. Remove from the oven and cool on a wire rack. The filling will be slightly runny but will thicken as it cools. SERVES 8

REDUCED-SUGAR COCONUT-PECAN PIE
Follow the directions for the Coconut-Pecan Pie (page 207), but reduce the sugar to ½ cup (100 g), add ⅛ teaspoon of stevia, and reduce the lemon juice to 1 tablespoon.

Coconut-Almond Pie

¼ cup (½ stick/55 g) salted butter, softened to room temperature
1 cup (200 g) sugar
2 large eggs
2 tablespoons (15 g) flour
½ cup (120 ml) coconut milk
¼ teaspoon almond extract
1½ cups (128 g) grated coconut
1 9-inch (23-cm) unbaked pastry shell
1 cup (100 g) sliced or slivered almonds

PREHEAT THE OVEN TO 350°F (180°C). In a large bowl, cream the butter and sugar until light. Add the eggs, one at a time, beating well after each addition. Sprinkle in the flour and blend until smooth. Mix in the coconut milk, almond extract, and grated coconut and spoon the mixture into the unbaked pastry shell. Sprinkle the almonds on top. Bake for about 45 minutes, until browned and springy to the touch. Cool on a wire rack and serve at room temperature. SERVES 8

REDUCED-SUGAR COCONUT-ALMOND PIE

Follow the directions for Coconut-Almond Pie (page 208), but reduce the sugar to ½ cup (100 g) and add ⅛ teaspoon of stevia.

Coconut-Peach Crisp

FILLING:

> 5 to 6 pitted, peeled, and sliced peaches
> 2 tablespoons (15 g) flour
> ½ teaspoon ground cinnamon
> ¼ cup (60 g) sucanat or firmly packed dark brown sugar

TOPPING:

> ¾ cup (60 g) old-fashioned oats
> ¾ cup (170 g) sucanat or firmly packed dark brown sugar
> ½ cup (62 g) flour
> ¾ cup (64 g) flaked coconut
> ½ cup (1 stick/112 g) unsalted butter or coconut oil, softened
> Dash of salt
> Coconut Whipped Cream (page 196), for topping

PREHEAT THE OVEN TO 400°F (200°C). For the filling, in a medium bowl, mix together the peaches, flour, cinnamon, and sucanat. Arrange the peach mixture in an 8 x 8 x 2-inch (20 x 20 x 5-cm) baking pan and set aside. For the topping, in a medium bowl, mix together the oats, sucanat, flour, coconut, butter, and salt and layer the mixture on top of the peaches. Bake for 30 minutes. Serve topped with Coconut Whipped Cream.   SERVES 6

COCONUT-APPLE CRISP

Make the Coconut-Peach Crisp (above) as directed, but substitute tart apples for the peaches.

REDUCED-SUGAR COCONUT-PEACH CRISP

Make the Coconut-Peach Crisp (above) as directed, but delete the sugar from the peach mixture. Reduce the sucanat in the topping to ¼ cup (60 g) and add ⅛ teaspoon of stevia.

Fruit and Coconut Cobbler

   1 cup (125 g) flour
   ½ cup (50 g) sugar
   ½ cup (42 g) grated coconut
   1½ teaspoons baking powder
   ¼ teaspoon salt
   ¼ cup (60 ml) coconut oil, melted
   ¼ cup (60 ml) coconut milk
   2 large eggs, slightly beaten
   Fruit filling Coconut Whipped Cream (page 196), for serving of your
       choice (recipes below)

PREHEAT THE OVEN TO 400°F (200°C). All of the ingredients should be at room temperature so that the coconut oil mixes evenly. In a large bowl, mix together the flour, sugar, coconut, baking powder, and salt. Add the coconut oil, coconut milk, and eggs and stir just to moisten. Spoon the dough on top of the fruit filling. Bake for 25 to 30 minutes, until golden. Cool and serve with Coconut Whipped Cream.   SERVES 6

Peach Filling

   ½ cup (100 g) sugar
   1 tablespoon (8 g) cornstarch
   ¼ teaspoon ground cinnamon
   1 teaspoon freshly squeezed lemon juice
   ½ cup (120 ml) peach juice or water
   4 cups (680 g) sliced fresh peaches

IN A BOWL, mix together the sugar, cornstarch, cinnamon, lemon juice, and peach juice. Add in the peaches and pour into a 11 x 7 x 1.5 inches (28 x 18 x 4 cm) baking dish. Top with the dough and cook as directed.   SERVES 6

CHERRY FILLING

Follow the directions for the Peach Filling (above), but substitute 4 cups (620 g) of pitted red tart cherries for the peaches and substitute ¼ teaspoon of almond extract for the lemon juice.

APPLE FILLING

Follow the directions for the Peach Filling (page 210), but substitute 4 cups (440 g) of sliced tart apples for the peaches and add ¼ teaspoon of ground nutmeg.

REDUCED-SUGAR COBBLER

Make the cobbler dough as directed in the Fruit and Coconut Cobbler (page 210), but reduce the sugar to 2 tablespoons (26 g) and add ⅛ teaspoon of powdered stevia. Reduce the sugar in the Peach Filling (above) and Apple Filling (above) to ¼ cup (50 g) or less. For the Cherry Filling (above), reduce the sugar to ½ cup (100 g) and use ¼ teaspoon of stevia in the batter.

Cream Puffs and Éclairs

Cream Puffs

½ cup (120 ml) water
¼ cup (½ stick/55 g) salted butter
Dash of salt
½ cup (62 g) flour
2 large eggs
Cream filling of your choice (recipes below)
Confectioners' sugar, for sprinkling

PREHEAT THE OVEN TO 400°F (200°C). In a small saucepan, add the water, butter, and salt and bring to a boil over high heat. Reduce the heat to low, add the flour all at once, and stir vigorously for about 1 minute, until the mixture forms a ball. Remove from the heat. Add the eggs all at once and continue beating until smooth. The mixture will look odd at first, almost like it's curdled, but as you beat, it will become smooth. Drop the dough by scant ¼ cupfuls about 3 inches (7.5 cm) apart onto an ungreased baking sheet. Bake for 35 to 40 minutes, until puffed and golden brown. Remove the puffs from the pan while still hot. Let cool on a wire rack. Cut off the tops. The puffs will be hollow. Fill the puffs with cream filling. Replace the tops and sprinkle with confectioners' sugar. Keep refrigerated and serve chilled.

MAKES 12 CREAM PUFFS

Cream Fillings

Vanilla Cream Filling

1 can (14 ounces/400 ml) coconut milk

⅓ cup (66 g) sugar

¼ cup (32 g) cornstarch

⅛ teaspoon salt

2 large egg yolks, slightly beaten

2 tablespoons (¼ stick/28 g) salted butter, softened

2 teaspoons vanilla extract

IN A LARGE SAUCEPAN, mix the coconut milk, sugar, cornstarch, and salt. Cook over medium heat, stirring constantly, until the mixture thickens. Boil and stir for 1 minute. Stir at least half of the hot mixture slowly into the egg yolks; stir the egg yolk mixture back into the hot mixture. Boil and stir for 1 minute. Remove from the heat; stir in the butter and vanilla. Allow the filling to cool.   MAKES ABOUT 2 CUPS

REDUCED-SUGAR CREAM FILLING

Make the Vanilla Cream Filling (above) as directed, but reduce the sugar to 2 tablespoons (26 g) and add a dash or two of stevia.

BANANA CREAM FILLING

Make the Vanilla Cream Filling (above) as directed, but reduce the sugar to 1 tablespoon (13 g) and add ½ cup (112 g) of ripe mashed banana with the butter and vanilla. For a reduced-sugar version, omit the sugar.

ALMOND CREAM FILLING

Make the Vanilla Cream Filling (above) as directed, but add 1 teaspoon of almond extract along with the vanilla.

CHOCOLATE CREAM FILLING

Make the Vanilla Cream Filling (page 212) as directed, but stir in 6 tablespoons (65 g) of semisweet chocolate chips into the mixture along with the butter and vanilla.

CARAMEL CREAM FILLING

Make the Vanilla Cream Filling (page 212) as directed, but substitute sucanat for the sugar.

LEMON CREAM FILLING

Make the Vanilla Cream Filling (page 212) as directed, but stir in ½ cup (120 ml) of freshly squeezed lemon juice into the mixture along with the butter and vanilla.

Chocolate Éclairs

MAKE THE CREAM puff dough as directed (Cream Puffs, page 211). Drop the dough by scant ¼ cupfuls onto an ungreased baking sheet. Using a spatula, shape each into a log 4½ inches (14 cm) long and 1½ inches (4 cm) wide. Bake and cool. Fill the puffs with cream filling. Cover with Chocolate Frosting (recipe below). Refrigerate and serve chilled.   MAKES 10 ÉCLAIRS

Chocolate Frosting

IN A SMALL SAUCEPAN, heat ½ square (½ ounce/14 g) of unsweetened chocolate and ½ teaspoon of unsalted butter over low heat until melted. Remove from the heat. Stir in ½ cup (60 g) of confectioners' sugar and about 1 tablespoon (15 ml) of hot water. Beat until smooth.

MAKES ABOUT ⅓ CUP FROSTING

PUDDINGS

Coconut-Vanilla Pudding

1 can (14 ounces/400 ml) coconut milk or coconut cream

2 tablespoons (16 g) cornstarch

½ cup (100 g) sugar

Dash of salt

1 tablespoon (14 g) salted butter

1 large egg, slightly beaten

2 teaspoons vanilla extract

Toasted flaked coconut

IN A MEDIUM SAUCEPAN, mix together the coconut milk, cornstarch, sugar, and salt. Put over medium heat, stirring constantly, until the mixture boils. Add the butter and boil and stir for 1 minute. Remove from the heat. In a small bowl, pour about 1 cup of the hot mixture, very slowly, into the egg, stirring constantly. Return the egg mixture to the pan. Cook and stir for 2 to 3 minutes, until no raw taste of egg remains. Do not boil. Remove from the heat. Stir in the vanilla and let cool slightly. Pour the pudding into custard cups. Serve hot or chilled, topped with toasted flaked coconut.   SERVES 2

CARAMEL PUDDING

Prepare the Coconut-Vanilla Pudding (above) as directed, but substitute ¾ cup (175 g) of firmly packed dark brown sugar or sucanat for the granulated sugar.

MAPLE PUDDING

Prepare the Coconut-Vanilla Pudding (page 215) as directed, but omit the sugar and replace it with maple sugar.

ALMOND PUDDING

Prepare the Coconut-Vanilla Pudding (page 215) as directed, but reduce the vanilla to 1 teaspoon and add ½ teaspoon of almond extract. Top with toasted sliced almonds.

REDUCED-SUGAR COCONUT-VANILLA PUDDING

Make the Coconut-Vanilla Pudding (page 215) as directed, but reduce the sugar to ¼ cup (50 g) and add a dash or two of powdered stevia.

Chocolate Pudding ⚙

3 tablespoons (16 g) cocoa powder
⅓ cup (66 g) sugar
Dash of salt
3 tablespoons (45 ml) water
1 can (14 ounces/400 ml) coconut milk or coconut cream
2 tablespoons (16 g) cornstarch
1 teaspoon vanilla extract
Coconut flakes or sliced almonds, toasted

IN A MEDIUM SAUCEPAN, mix together the cocoa, sugar, and salt; stir in the water. Cook and stir over medium heat until the mixture boils; boil and stir for 2 minutes. In a medium bowl using a handheld mixer, mix together the coconut milk and cornstarch until blended, or use a wire whisk and whisk until blended. Pour the coconut milk mixture into the hot mixture, stirring constantly. Continue to cook for 5 or 6 minutes, until the mixture thickens. Remove from the heat and blend in the vanilla. Cool and pour into custard cups. Serve hot or cold. Top with toasted coconut flakes or toasted sliced almonds just before serving.   SERVES 2

HALF AND HALF PUDDING ⚙

Make the Coconut-Vanilla Pudding (page 215), fill custard cups halfway, and chill. Make the Chocolate Pudding (page 216) and let cool. Pour the Chocolate Pudding into the center of the Coconut Vanilla Pudding (do not stir) and chill until set. Before serving, top with toasted flaked coconut or sliced almonds.

Banana Pudding ⚙

> 2 medium bananas, thinly sliced
> 1 can (14 ounces/400 ml) coconut milk
> ½ teaspoon ground cinnamon
> 1 teaspoon honey
> Dash of salt
> Shredded coconut, toasted

IN A MEDIUM SAUCEPAN, combine the bananas, coconut milk, cinnamon, honey, and salt and bring to a boil over high heat. Reduce the heat to medium-low and simmer for about 8 minutes, until the mixture thickens and the banana partially dissolves. Let cool. This pudding can be eaten warm or cold. As it cools, the pudding thickens. Serve with toasted coconut sprinkled on top.   SERVES 2

Coconut Pudding Squares

This is a rich, sweet, gelatinous dessert that is popular in Hawaii.

> 1 can (14 ounces/400 ml) coconut milk
> 7 tablespoons (91 g) sugar
> 7 tablespoons (56 g) cornstarch
> Dash of salt

IN A MEDIUM SAUCEPAN, mix the coconut milk, sugar, cornstarch, and salt. Bring to a boil over high heat; reduce the heat to low and simmer, stirring constantly, until the mixture thickens. Keep stirring over low heat until the mixture becomes very thick and sticky. Pour into an 8 x 8 x 2-inch pan and chill until firm. Cut into 2-inch squares and serve.   **MAKES 16 SQUARES**

Brown Rice Pudding

> ½ cup (95 g) uncooked brown rice (see Note)
> ½ cup (120 ml) water
> 1 can (14 ounces/400 ml) coconut milk
> 1 tablespoon (20 g) honey
> 2 or 3 dashes of salt

IN A MEDIUM SAUCEPAN, soak the brown rice in the water for at least 4 hours or overnight. Add the coconut milk, honey, and salt; bring to a boil over high heat. Reduce the heat to low, cover, and simmer for about 40 minutes, until the rice is soft and most, but not all, of the liquid is absorbed. Serve hot. This makes a great lightly sweetened dessert or breakfast.

SERVES 2

Note

This recipe can be made with white rice if you prefer. If you use white rice, reduce the cooking time to about 20 minutes.

VANILLA RICE PUDDING

Follow the directions for Brown Rice Pudding (above), but add 2 teaspoons of vanilla extract after the rice has been cooked.

ALMOND RICE PUDDING

Follow the directions for Brown Rice Pudding (above), but add 1 teaspoon of almond extract and ½ cup (55 g) of toasted slivered almonds after the rice has been cooked.

RICE PUDDING WITH FRESH FRUIT

This recipe goes well mixed with fresh sliced fruit. Add the fruit to the rice after it is cooked. Fruits that go well include peaches, mangos, bananas, strawberries, blueberries, boysenberries, blackberries, raspberries, and pineapple.

CINNAMON-APPLE RICE PUDDING

Follow the directions for Brown Rice Pudding (page 218), but add 1 teaspoon of cinnamon and 1 chopped tart apple to the rice before cooking.

CINNAMON-RAISIN RICE PUDDING

Follow the directions for Brown Rice Pudding (page 218), but add 1 teaspoon of cinnamon and ½ cup (75 g) of raisins to the rice before cooking.

Baked Custard

> 3 large eggs
> 1 can (14 ounces/400 ml) coconut milk
> ⅓ cup (66 g) sugar
> Dash of salt
> 1 teaspoon vanilla extract
> Ground nutmeg

PREHEAT THE OVEN TO 350°F (180°C). In a medium bowl, lightly beat together the eggs, coconut milk, sugar, salt, and vanilla. Pour into six 6-ounce (175-ml) custard cups; sprinkle the tops with nutmeg. Place the cups in a baking pan about 13 x 9 x 2 inches (33 x 23 x 50 cm) in size. Pour very hot water into the pan up to ½ inch (13 mm) from the tops of the custard cups. Bake for 45 minutes, or until a knife inserted in the custard comes out clean. Remove the cups from the water and serve warm or chilled.   SERVES 6

MAPLE CUSTARD

Prepare the Baked Custard (above) as directed, but substitute maple sugar for the sugar.

REDUCED-SUGAR CUSTARD

Prepare the Baked Custard (above) as directed, but reduce the sugar to 3 tablespoons (39 g) and add a dash or two of stevia.

Tapioca

½ cup (76 g) quick-cooking tapioca
3 cups (495 ml) coconut milk
½ cup (100 g) sugar
¼ teaspoon salt
2 large eggs, beaten
1 teaspoon vanilla extract

IN A LARGE SAUCEPAN, heat the tapioca, coconut milk, sugar, and salt over high heat. Bring to a boil, stirring constantly. Reduce the heat to low and simmer for 8 to 10 minutes, uncovered. In a small bowl, slowly stir half of the hot tapioca into the beaten eggs, then combine the eggs with the other half of the hot mixture. Simmer, stirring constantly, until thickened. Remove from the heat, add the vanilla, and cool. Serve warm or chilled.
MAKES ABOUT 3 CUPS

CHOCOLATE TAPIOCA

Make the Tapioca (above) as directed, but add 2 ounces (58 g) of unsweetened chocolate.

REDUCED-SUGAR TAPIOCA

Make the Tapioca (above) according to the directions, but reduce the sugar to ¼ cup (50 g) and add a dash or two of powdered stevia.

Fruity Tapioca Pudding

½ cup (100 g) sugar
¼ cup (38 g) quick-cooking tapioca
1¾ cups (410 ml) freshly squeezed orange juice
¾ cup (175 ml) coconut milk
Dash of salt
¼ cup (35 g) raisins or cut-up dates
1 orange, sectioned and cut into bite-size pieces
¼ cup (21 g) flaked coconut

IN A LARGE SAUCEPAN, mix together the sugar, tapioca, orange juice, coconut milk, and salt. Let stand for 5 minutes. Heat to a boil over high heat, reduce the heat to medium-low, and simmer for 8 minutes, stirring constantly. Remove from the heat and add the raisins. Cool slightly. Stir in the orange sections. Refrigerate for at least 1 hour. Sprinkle the top with coconut and serve.   SERVES 4

REDUCED-SUGAR FRUITY TAPIOCA PUDDING
Make the Fruity Tapioca Pudding (page 220) as directed, but omit the sugar and add ⅛ teaspoon of powdered stevia.

ICE CREAM

Homemade Ice Cream

If you like coconut and you like ice cream, this chapter will be one of your favorites. The best way to make homemade ice cream is with an ice cream maker. Because not everyone has an ice cream maker, I am including directions on how to make ice cream using a blender. The blender method makes a relatively smooth, delicious-tasting ice cream. Ice cream makers, however, produce a much smoother, lighter product that is superior in taste and texture. If you plan on making a lot of ice cream—and you may once you try some of these recipes—I recommend buying an ice cream maker. They don't really cost that much and are well worth the price.

Basic Ice Cream Recipes

You can choose from three basic vanilla ice cream recipes: Quick, Premium, and Reduced-Sugar. All of the ice cream flavors described in this chapter can be made using any of these three basic recipes. The Quick recipe, as the name implies, is the simplest and easiest to make. The Premium recipe is made using eggs; it takes a little longer and requires a bit more care but produces a smoother-textured product that more closely resembles commercial ice cream. The Reduced-Sugar recipe is for those people who want to enjoy the creamy richness and flavor of ice cream without all of the sugar.

Because the three basic recipes are made using coconut milk or coconut cream rather than dairy milk, they are each referred to as *Coconut*-Vanilla Ice Cream rather than just vanilla ice cream. The coconut milk gives them a slightly different but great-tasting flavor. Coconut-Vanilla Ice Cream is used as the basis for all of the flavors described in this chapter. Use whichever one of the three you want in making the various flavors that follow.

Homemade ice cream generally freezes a little harder than commercial ice cream. When first taken out of the freezer, it can be a bit difficult to scoop out. If you let it sit at room temperature for about 10 or 15 minutes, it will be much easier to work with.

Quick Coconut-Vanilla Ice Cream

> 1 can (14 ounces/400 ml) coconut milk or cream
> 2 tablespoons (26 g) sugar
> Dash of salt
> 1 tablespoon (15 ml) vanilla extract

IN A SMALL SAUCEPAN, combine the coconut milk, sugar, and salt. Cook over low to medium heat until the ingredients are dissolved. Do not boil. Remove from the heat and stir in the vanilla. If you have an ice cream maker, put the mixture in the refrigerator until chilled. Follow the directions given with your unit.

If you do not have an ice cream maker, pour the mixture into a freezer-safe container and freeze. A convenient container is an ice cube tray. Freeze the mixture for about 2 hours, until it is mostly, but not completely, solid. If the mixture becomes completely frozen, take it out of the freezer and let it sit at room temperature until it begins to melt. You want the mixture to be cold (about 32°F/0°C) but not frozen solid. In the bowl of a blender, place the mixture and blend at high speed. If the mixture is too hard, it will not blend well; wait for it to warm up a little and try again. While blending, the mixture should take on the appearance and texture of a thick milk shake. Eat immediately or pour the ice cream into an airtight container and freeze. Blending the mixture and freezing it a second time like this crushes the ice crystals that form during the first freezing and gives the ice cream a smoother, creamier texture.   SERVES 2

Premium Coconut-Vanilla Ice Cream

> 1 can (14 ounces/400 ml) coconut milk or coconut cream
> ¼ cup (60 ml) coconut oil (optional) (see Note)
> 2½ tablespoons (32 g) sugar
> Dash of salt
> 1 large egg
> 1 tablespoon (15 ml) vanilla extract

IN A MEDIUM SAUCEPAN, combine the coconut milk, coconut oil, sugar, and salt. Cook over medium heat, stirring occasionally, until the mixture almost boils. Reduce the heat to low. In a small bowl, beat the egg. Gradually stir about ½ cup (120 ml) of the hot coconut milk into the beaten egg. Slowly stir this egg mixture into the remaining hot coconut milk. Cook over low heat, stirring constantly, for 2 to 3 minutes, until slightly thickened. Stir in the vanilla. Remove from the heat and let cool. Use the blender or ice cream maker method to finish.   SERVES 2

Note
Coconut oil gives the ice cream a richer, creamier taste and texture, especially if you use coconut milk. It can be omitted if you use coconut cream.

REDUCED-SUGAR COCONUT-VANILLA ICE CREAM
Follow the directions for making either Quick Coconut-Vanilla Ice Cream (page 224) or Premium Coconut-Vanilla Ice Cream (above), but reduce the sugar to 4 teaspoons or less and add a dash or two of stevia.   SERVES 2

Ice Cream Flavors

Use any of the three basic Coconut-Vanilla Ice Cream recipes (pages 224, 225) for the flavors described below. Unless otherwise noted, use one full recipe of Coconut-Vanilla Ice Cream as the basis for all of other flavors. The basic recipes make 2 to 3 cups (280 to 420 g) of ice cream, depending on the method and version you use. Ice cream makers stir air into the mixture, giving the ice cream greater volume. The Premium Coconut-Vanilla Ice Cream (page 225) made using an ice cream maker produces the best results for all flavors.

Double-Coconut Ice Cream

1 full recipe Coconut-Vanilla Ice Cream (pages 224 to 225)
1 teaspoon imitation coconut extract (optional)
¼ cup (21 g) flaked coconut, toasted

MAKE THE COCONUT-VANILLA Ice Cream according to the directions, adding the imitation coconut extract along with the vanilla. Just before serving, garnish with toasted flaked coconut.   SERVES 2

Coconut-Pineapple Ice Cream

1 full recipe Coconut-Vanilla Ice Cream (pages 224 to 225)
1¼ cups (206 g) crushed pineapple with juice
⅓ cup (28 g) flaked coconut

MAKE THE COCONUT-VANILLA Ice Cream according to the directions. Place the pineapple in the refrigerator for at least 1 hour, to chill. After removing the ice cream from the ice cream maker or blender, add the chilled crushed pineapple and mix thoroughly. Put immediately into the freezer to harden.

Preheat the oven to 350°F (180°C). Place the flaked coconut on a baking sheet or in a glass baking pan. Spread the flakes out to make an even layer. Bake in the oven for about 10 minutes, or until golden brown. Just before serving the ice cream, sprinkle the top with the toasted coconut. Use freshly toasted coconut for best results.   SERVES 2

Orange Cream Delight ⊛

> **1 full recipe Coconut-Vanilla Ice Cream (pages 224 to 225)**
> **1¼ cups (295 ml) freshly squeezed orange juice**

MAKE THE COCONUT-VANILLA Ice Cream according to the directions. Before adding the mixture to the ice cream maker or blender, combine with the orange juice. This recipe makes a delicious, creamy orange-flavored ice cream.   SERVES 2

CHOCOLATE-ORANGE DELIGHT ⊛
Follow the directions for the Orange Cream Delight (above) and freeze. Before serving, drizzle chocolate syrup on top. Enjoy!

Fruit Sherbet

This recipe makes a delicious, sherbet-like fruit-flavored ice cream.

> **1 full recipe Coconut-Vanilla Ice Cream (pages 224 to 225)**
> **1¾ to 2 cups (410 to 475 ml) fruit juice**

MAKE THE COCONUT-VANILLA Ice Cream according to the directions. When the ice cream mixture is taken off the stove, add the fruit juice. Different brands of juice vary in flavor and sweetness, so taste the mixture and add more juice or sugar to suit your taste. Finish by using the blender or ice cream maker method.

Almost any kind of fruit juice will work in this recipe. Stores, and particularly health food stores, carry a wide selection of bottled and frozen fruit juices. Some of the juices I've seen include orange, lime, lemon, peach, papaya, guava, mango, apricot, cherry, cranberry, raspberry, orange mango, blueberry, grape, cranberry grape, pineapple, and even coconut nectar. Some juices are very sweet and you may want to reduce the sugar in the original recipe to 1 tablespoon (13 g) or less and adjust the sweetness after you add the juice. SERVES 4

Fruit-Flavored Ice Cream

This makes a delicious, creamy, fruit-flavored ice cream. This recipe has less water than the Fruit Sherbet (page 227), allowing the finished product to have a higher percentage of coconut cream. Almost any flavor of frozen fruit juice concentrate works with this recipe.

> 1 full recipe Coconut-Vanilla Ice Cream (pages 224 to 225)
> ½ cup (about 150 g) frozen fruit juice concentrate, no water added

MAKE THE COCONUT-VANILLA Ice Cream according to the directions. When all of the ingredients have been combined on the stove, remove the mixture from the heat and let cool. While cooling, add the frozen fruit juice concentrate, without added water. Let it melt and mix thoroughly. Finish by using the blender or ice cream maker method. SERVES 2

Coconut Sherbet

This very simple and easy sherbet is made with young coconut water rather than coconut milk or coconut cream. For best results, use coconut water from immature or green coconuts rather than the juice from a mature coconut. If you don't have access to fresh young coconuts, you can use commercially produced coconut water.

All you need for this sherbet is coconut water and an ice cream maker. Let the ice cream maker churn and freeze the water into a sherbet, just as you would any other sherbet. There is no need to add sugar or anything else. The end product is a delicious-tasting coconut sherbet.

MAKES 1 SERVING PER COCONUT

Strawberry Ice Cream ⚙

> 1 full recipe Coconut-Vanilla Ice Cream (pages 224 to 225)
> 1½ to 2 cups (220 to 290 g) fresh or frozen strawberries

MAKE THE COCONUT-VANILLA Ice Cream as described, but increase the sugar to 3 tablespoons (39 g). Before freezing or putting the mixture into an ice cream maker, add the strawberries and blend in a blender. Taste for sweetness and add more sugar if needed. Finish by using the ice cream maker or blender method.   SERVES 3 TO 4

FRESH FRUIT ICE CREAM

A variety of fruit ice creams can be made using the Strawberry Ice Cream (above) recipe but with different fresh fruits. Some good ones include raspberries, blackberries, blueberries, cherries, and peaches. Ripeness and sweetness vary, so you may need to adjust the sugar content.

Chunky Chocolate-Almond Ice Cream ⚙

> 1 cup (145 g) whole or chopped almonds
> 5 tablespoons (94 g) chocolate syrup
> 1 full recipe Coconut-Vanilla Ice Cream (pages 224 to 225)
> 1 teaspoon almond extract

PREHEAT THE OVEN TO 325°F (170°C). Place the almonds on a rimmed baking sheet and toast for 10 to 15 minutes, or until slightly browned. In a small bowl, stir the toasted almonds into the chocolate and set aside to cool. Make the Coconut-Vanilla Ice Cream recipe according to directions, but add the almond extract at the same time as the vanilla. The chocolate almond mixture should be at room temperature or cooler before adding it to the ice cream. Just before placing the ice cream in the freezer, add the chocolate almond mixture, a spoonful at a time. Stir several times to evenly distribute the chocolate and almond chunks; then freeze the mixture.
SERVES 3

Peppermint Ice Cream

1 full recipe Coconut-Vanilla Ice Cream (pages 224 to 225)
1 teaspoon peppermint extract
0.4 ounce (13 g) crushed peppermint candy (optional)

MAKE THE COCONUT-VANILLA ICE CREAM recipe according to the directions, but add the peppermint extract at the same time as the vanilla. After the ice cream is churned and just before freezing, mix in the crushed peppermint candy.   SERVES 2

Maple-Nut Ice Cream

1 full recipe Coconut-Vanilla Ice Cream (pages 224 to 225)
3 tablespoons (60 g) maple syrup
¼ cup (30 g) chopped walnuts or black walnuts

MAKE THE COCONUT-VANILLA ICE CREAM according to the directions, substituting the maple syrup for the sugar. Just before freezing, mix in the chopped nuts.   SERVES 2

Chocolate Ice Cream (Basic Recipe)

This is a basic recipe you can use for any variety of chocolate ice cream.

¼ cup (60 ml) coconut oil
3 tablespoons (16 g) cocoa powder
1¾ cups (410 ml) coconut milk or coconut cream
Dash of salt
⅓ cup (66 g) sugar
1 tablespoon (15 ml) vanilla extract

IN A SMALL SAUCEPAN, melt the coconut oil over low heat. Add the cocoa and mix thoroughly. Keep the cocoa mixture on low heat, stirring frequently; be careful not to boil. In a second saucepan, heat the coconut milk, salt, and sugar over medium heat until the sugar is completely dissolved. With the cocoa mixture on low heat, slowly pour the coconut milk mixture into it while stirring. Continue to stir until the mixtures blend, forming a smooth, creamy chocolate. Add the vanilla. Finish by using the ice cream maker or blender method. SERVES 2

QUICK CHOCOLATE ICE CREAM

A quick and easy method of making chocolate ice cream is to add ⅓ cup (100 g) of chocolate syrup to the Coconut-Vanilla Ice Cream (pages 224 to 225) before putting it into the ice cream maker.

Rocky Road Ice Cream ✿

> 1 full recipe Chocolate Ice Cream (Basic Recipe) (page 230)
> ¾ cup (38 g) miniature marshmallows
> ½ cup (about 55 g) chopped nuts

MAKE THE CHOCOLATE ICE CREAM (Basic Recipe) according to the directions. Before putting the ice cream into the freezer, stir in the marshmallows and nuts. SERVES 3

Chocolate-Marshmallow Swirl Ice Cream ✿

> ¾ cup (108 g) whole or chopped almonds
> 1 full recipe Chocolate Ice Cream (Basic Recipe) (page 230)
> 1 cup (226 g) marshmallow cream

PREHEAT THE OVEN TO 325°F (170°C). Place the almonds on a rimmed baking sheet and toast them in the oven for 10 to 15 minutes, or until slightly browned. Set aside to cool. Make the Chocolate Ice Cream recipe according to the directions. Before freezing the ice cream, add the marshmallow cream and the toasted almonds and stir them in just enough to create a swirl effect. SERVES 3

Toffee–Chocolate Chip Ice Cream

> 1 full recipe Coconut-Vanilla Ice Cream (pages 224 to 225)
> ½ teaspoon almond extract
> ⅓ cup (93 g) English toffee bits
> ½ cup (88 g) milk chocolate chips

MAKE THE COCONUT-VANILLA ICE CREAM according to the directions and add the almond extract with the vanilla. Before putting the mixture into the freezer, mix in the toffee bits and chocolate chips.   SERVES 2

Fried Ice Cream ✿

The secret to fried ice cream is in the making of the crust. The crust in this recipe consists of toasted almonds and coconut. Sliced almonds work best, but you may use slivered or even chopped almonds. Unlike what the name implies, this ice cream isn't actually fried. It is coated in a layer of toasted almonds and coconut. Traditionally vanilla ice cream is used, but strawberry or chocolate ice cream also tastes great.

> 1 full recipe Coconut-Vanilla Ice Cream (pages 224 to 225)
> ½ cup (48 g) sliced almonds
> ½ cup (42 g) coconut flakes
> ¼ cup (85 g) honey

MAKE THE COCONUT-VANILLA ICE CREAM according to the directions and freeze for at least 3 hours. Before serving, preheat the oven to 325°F (170°C). Place the almonds and coconut flakes in a single layer on a rimmed baking sheet and bake in the oven for about 10 minutes, or until the coconut is golden brown. Remove from the oven and cool. Scoop the ice cream out in serving-size balls. Roll the balls in the toasted coating or simply sprinkle the coating on the ice cream. Use a generous amount of coating; sprinkle the remaining coating along the sides of serving bowls. Drizzle a little honey on top and serve.   SERVES 2

Creamy Fudge Ice Cream

This ice cream tastes just like the Fudgsicles from the store.

¼ cup (50 g) sugar
2 tablespoons (11 g) cocoa powder
Dash of salt
3 tablespoons (45 ml) water
1 can (14 ounces/400 ml) coconut milk or coconut cream
½ teaspoon vanilla extract

IN A MEDIUM SAUCEPAN, mix together the sugar, cocoa, and salt; stir in the water. Stir over medium heat until the mixture boils and the sugar dissolves. Stir in the coconut milk. Remove from the heat; add the vanilla. Let cool. Store in the freezer. SERVES 2

Frozen Chocolate Bananas

2 bananas, halved crosswise
4 wooden sticks
1 package (6 ounces/131 g) semisweet chocolate chips
2 tablespoons (30 ml) coconut oil
½ cup (42 g) flaked coconut, toasted

LINE A BAKING sheet or plate with wax paper. Insert wooden sticks into the banana halves, place on the wax paper, and put in the freezer overnight or until frozen. In a small, heavy saucepan, melt the chocolate and coconut oil over low heat, stirring constantly. When melted, remove from the heat and let cool to room temperature. The mixture should still be soft. Remove the bananas from freezer and dip them into the chocolate, spreading the chocolate to form a fairly even coating. Immediately roll in the toasted coconut and place back on the wax paper. Freeze for at least 30 minutes. If not eaten that day, store in an airtight container. SERVES 4

INDEX

Page numbers in **bold** indicate tables.

Africa, 3
African Coconut Shrimp, 113
almonds
  Almond Chicken Stir-Fry, 96–97
  Almond Chicken with Noodles, 104
  Almond-Coconut Cookies, 186
  Almond Cream Filling, Cream
    Puffs, 212
  Almond Oil, 69
  Almond Pudding, 215, 216
  Almond Rice Pudding, 218
  Almond Whipped Cream, 196–97
  Chicken Amandine, 101
  Chocolate Almond, 25–26
  Chunky Chocolate-Almond Ice
    Cream, 229
  Coconut-Almond Macaroons, 177, 178
  Coconut-Almond Pie, 208–9
Ambrosia, 48
apples
  Ambrosia, 48
  Apple and Sweet Potato Curry,
    125–26
  Apple-Cinnamon Salad, 51
  Apple-Coconut Cake, 170–71
  Apple Filling for Cobbler, 210, 211
  Applesauce Cake, 168–69
  Carrot-Apple Curry, 52
  Cinnamon-Apple Coconut Cake,
    175–76
  Cinnamon-Apple Rice Pudding,
    218, 219
  Coconut-Apple Crisp, 209
  Peanut Butter–Apple Slaw, 53
  Waldorf Salad, 48
Apricot-Coconut Bars, 187
Apricot Milk, 23
Artichoke Soup, Cream of, 77–78
artificial sweeteners, 16
Asia, 2
Asian-style cuisine, 115–34
Asparagus and Shrimp and Coconut
    Sauce, 113–14
Asparagus Soup, Cream of, 75
Ayurvedic medicine, 3

Bacon and Cheese Potatoes, 136, 137
Baked Blueberry Pancake, 152
Baked Custard, 219
Baked Peach Pancake, 152
Baked Potato, Super, 137
Baked Single-Crust Pie Shell, 195
Baked (Twice) Potato, 137–38
bananas
  Ambrosia, 48
  Banana-Coconut Cake, 168
  Banana-Coconut Salad, 49
  Banana Cream Filling, Cream
    Puffs, 212
  Banana Cream Pie, 199, 200

bananas (*cont.*)
  Banana Milk, 23
  Banana Pudding, 217
  Coconut-Banana Bread with Lime
    Glaze, 159–60
  Coconut-Banana Pancakes, 151–52
  Frozen Chocolate Bananas, 233
  Hawaiian Banana Bread, 161
  Orange-Banana Salad, 50
  Orange-Coconut Banana Bread,
    161–62
  Piña Colada Smoothie, 35
  Pineapple-Banana Milk, 24
  Raspberry-Banana Salad, 49–50
  Strawberry-Banana Smoothie, 40
  Zesty Mango-Banana Salad, 52
bars. *See* cookies
Basic Coconut Milk Smoothie, 32–33
Basic Ice Cream Recipes, 223–25
Basic Vanilla Cream Filling, 173–74
beef
  Beef Macaroni and Cheese, 142
  Beef Stir-Fry, 95–96
  Beef Stroganoff, 101–2
  Beefy Cheese Soup, 91–92
  Shepherd's Pie, 111
  Tamale Soup, 92–93
  Vegetable-Beef Potpie, 98–99
beverages, 1, 19–41
biscuits
  Cheese Biscuits, 158
  Coconut Milk Biscuits, 157
  Creamy Chicken and Biscuits, 109
  Creamy Tuna and Biscuits, 109–10
  Double Cheese Biscuits, 158
Black-Bottom–Custard Pie, 203–4
bladder infections, 2, 4
blender drinks. *See* smoothies and
    blender drinks
blueberries
  Baked Blueberry Pancake, 152
  Blueberry-Coconut Cake, 170–71
  Blueberry-Coconut Muffins, 147
  Blueberry Milk, 23
body fat loss, 4–5
Bran-Coconut Muffins, 145–46
breads and grains, 17, 145–63
breast milk, 4, 5
Broccoli and Creamy Cheese Soup,
    90–91
Broccoli Soup, Cream of, 75–76
Brown Rice Pudding, 218

Burmese Peanut Chicken, 134
Butter Coconut Cookies, 191–92
Buttermilk Dressing, 44
Butternut Soup, 93–94
Butternut Squash, Mashed, 138
Butter Orange Frosting, 181
Butterscotch Haystacks, 188

cakes, 165–76
calories in coconut, 5
Calypso Turkey Salad, 56–57
candidiasis, 4
canned coconut milk, 13, 14, 19, 197
Cantaloupe-Cherry Salad, 50–51
Caramel Cream Filling for Cream Puffs,
    212, 213
Caramel Cream Pie, 199, 200
Caramel Pudding, 215
carbohydrates in coconut, 2, 10–11
Cardamom Dressing, Creamy, 46
Cardamom Rice, 141
Caribbean, 3–4
Carrot-Apple Curry, 52
Carrot-Coconut Cake, 169–70
Carrot-Coconut Cookies, 181
casseroles, 1
  Chicken Rice Casserole, 107–8
  Ham and Potato Casserole, 110
  Spinach, Ham, and Potato
    Casserole, 110
  Tuna Noodle Casserole, 102
  Tuna Rice Casserole, 107–8
Catfish in Coconut Sauce, 106–7
Cauliflower and Shrimp in Coconut
    Sauce, 122–23
Cauliflower Soup, Cream of, 76
Cauliflower Soup, Curried Cream of, 77
Central America, 3
Cheddar Cheese Sauce, Thick, 63
Cheddar Cheese Tex-Mex Sauce, 63
cheese
  Bacon and Cheese Potatoes, 136, 137
  Beefy Cheese Soup, 91–92
  Cheese and Potato Soup, 91
  Cheese Biscuits, 158
  Cheese Cups, 2, 142–43
  Cheese Nachos, 144
  Cheesy Mashed Potatoes, 136
  Creamy Cheese and Broccoli Soup,
    90–91
  Double Cheese Biscuits, 158
  Macaroni and Cheese, 142

cheese sauces, 62–64
See also sauces
cherries
  Cantaloupe-Cherry Salad, 50–51
  Cherry-Coconut Muffins, 147
  Cherry Filling for Cobbler, 210
  Cherry-Yogurt Smoothie, 34
chicken
  Almond Chicken Stir-Fry, 96–97
  Almond Chicken with Noodles, 104
  Burmese Peanut Chicken, 134
  Chicken à La King, 2, 108
  Chicken Amandine, 101
  Chicken and Dumplings, 73–74
  Chicken and Rice Stew, 89
  Chicken and Sweet Potato Stew with
    Coconut Dumplings, 133–34
  Chicken and Vegetables in Cream
    Sauce, 120–21
  Chicken Gravy, 65–66
  Chicken in Curry Sauce, 119–20
  Chicken in Red Curry Sauce, 126
  Chicken Linguine, 99
  Chicken Potpie, 97–98
  Chicken Rice Casserole, 107–8
  Chicken Stir-Fry, 95–96
  Chunky Chicken Gravy, 67
  Coconut-Chicken Soup, 132
  Creamy Chicken and Biscuits, 109
  Hearty Chicken Stew, 74
  Indian-Style Chicken Stew, 118–19
  Orange-Coconut Chicken, 103
  Peanut Chicken, 125
  Potato and Pea Korma, 123–24
  Sesame Chicken, 103–4
  Sesame Chicken Salad, 2, 55
  Thai Chicken, 117–18
  Thai Chicken and Shrimp Soup, 94
Chiffon Pies, 200–203
Chips, Coconut Tortilla Corn, 144
chocolate
  Black-Bottom–Custard Pie, 203–4
  Chocolate Almond, 25–26
  Chocolate Chiffon Pie, 202–3
  Chocolate-Coconut Bars, 184–85
  Chocolate-Coconut Cream Filling,
    173–74
  Chocolate–Coconut-Oatmeal
    Cookies, 182–83
  Chocolate Cream Filling for Cream
    Puffs, 212, 213
  Chocolate Cream Pie, 199, 200

Chocolate Crisps/Crispies, 189–90
Chocolate Éclairs, 213
Chocolate Frosting, 213
Chocolate Fruit Smoothie, 34–35
Chocolate Granola Bars, 191
Chocolate Haystacks, 188
Chocolate Ice Cream, 230–31
Chocolate Macaroons, 177, 178
Chocolate-Marshmallow Swirl Ice
  Cream, 231
Chocolate Mint, 26
Chocolate-Orange Delight, 227
Chocolate Peanut Butter Smoothie, 35
Chocolate Pudding, 216
Chocolate Tapioca, 220
Chocolate Whipped Cream, 196–97
Chunky Chocolate-Almond Ice
  Cream, 229
Creamy Fudge Ice Cream, 233
Frozen Chocolate Bananas, 233
Frozen Chocolate-Coconut Pie,
  198–99
German Chocolate Cake, 166–67
Hot Chocolate, 25
Nutty Chocolate Chip Cookies, 179
Quick Chocolate Ice Cream, 231
Toffee–Chocolate Chip Ice Cream, 232
choosing a good coconut, 7–8
chowders, 1
  Corn and Potato Chowder, 86
  Corn Chowder, 85–86
  Crab Chowder, 84–85
  Deluxe Clam Chowder, 83
  Fish Chowder, 83
  New England Clam Chowder, 82
  Shrimp Chowder, 84
  See also soups and chowders
chronic fatigue, 2
Chunky Chicken Gravy, 67
Chunky Chocolate-Almond Ice
  Cream, 229
cinnamon
  Apple-Cinnamon Salad, 51
  Cinnamon-Apple Coconut Cake,
    175–76
  Cinnamon-Apple Rice Pudding,
    218, 219
  Cinnamon Eggnog, 27
  Cinnamon-Nut Muffins, 147–48
  Cinnamon-Raisin Rice Pudding,
    218, 219
  Creamy Cinnamon Dressing, 46

Citrus Cream Filling, 173–74
Citrus Refresher, 35–36
Clam Chowder, Deluxe, 83
Clam Chowder, New England, 82
Cobbler, Fruit and Coconut, 210–11
Cocktails, 29–31
coconut, cooking with, 1–15
　calories, 5
　canned coconut milk, 13, 14, 19, 197
　carbohydrates in coconut, 2, 10–11
　choosing a good coconut, 7–8
　coconut cream, 6, 7, 12, 13, 19, 197
　coconut flour, 10
　coconut meat, 2, 3, 6, **6,** 7, 9, 10–11
　coconut milk, 2, 3, 6, **6,** 7, 12–13, 17,
　　19–21
　coconut milk beverage, 13
　coconut oil, 1, 2, 3–6, **6,** 7, 10, 14–15,
　　36–38
　coconut water, 2–3, 6, 7, 11–12, 21–22
　cracked coconuts, 7–8
　cream of coconut, 12
　dried coconut (shredded, grated,
　　flaked), **6,** 9, 11, 17
　electrolytes in coconut water, 3, 12
　emulsifier for adding coconut oil,
　　37–38
　"eyes" of coconut, 8
　fat in coconut, 3, 5, 12, 13
　fiber in coconut (dietary fiber), 2,
　　10–11
　gluten sensitivity, 10
　health food (superior), 1, 2–5,
　　36, 37, 38
　low-carbohydrate diets, 2, 10–11
　medium-chain triglycerides (MCTs),
　　3, 4, 5
　melting point of coconut oil, 14, 37
　moldy coconuts, 7, 8
　opening a coconut, 8
　protein, 10
　recommended amount of coconut oil,
　　5–6, **6,** 36–37
　smoking point of coconut oil, 14
　storage, 8, 9, 13, 14, 19
　vegetable oils vs. coconut oil, 14
　white spots in coconuts, 7–8
Coconut-Almond Cookies, 186
Coconut-Almond Macaroons, 177, 178
Coconut-Almond Pie, 208–9
Coconut and Fruit Cobbler, 210–11
Coconut-Apple Cake, 170–71

Coconut-Apple Crisp, 209
Coconut-Apricot Bars, 187
Coconut-Banana Bread with Lime
　Glaze, 159–60
Coconut-Banana Cake, 168
Coconut-Banana Pancakes, 151–52
Coconut-Banana Salad, 49
Coconut Battered Shrimp, 111–12
Coconut-Blueberry Cake, 170–71
Coconut-Blueberry Muffins, 147
Coconut-Bran Muffins, 145–46
Coconut Butter Cookies, 192
Coconut Cake, 165–66
Coconut-Carrot Cake, 169–70
Coconut-Carrot Cookies, 181
Coconut-Cherry Muffins, 147
Coconut-Chicken Soup, 132
Coconut-Chocolate Bars, 184–85
Coconut-Chocolate Cream Filling,
　173–74
Coconut-Chocolate–Oatmeal Cookies,
　182–83
Coconut-Chocolate Pie, Frozen,
　198–99
Coconut Cinnamon-Apple Cake,
　175–76
Coconut–Corn Bread Muffins, 149
coconut cream, 6, 7, 12, 13, 19, 197
Coconut Cream Cake, 173–74
Coconut Cream Cake Filling, 173–74
Coconut Cream Pie, 2, 199, 200
Coconut Cream Sauce, 105
Coconut Custard Pie, 204
Coconut Custard Sauce, 62
Coconut-Double Ice Cream, 226
Coconut Dressing, Creamy, 46
Coconut Dumplings, 133–34
coconut flour, 10
Coconut Fruit Rice, 156
Coconut Fruity Pancakes, 150
Coconut Jumbo Fried Shrimp, 112
Coconut Ketogenic Diet, The (Fife), 5
Coconut Kisses, 178–79
Coconut-Lime Pie, 206
Coconut Macaroons, 2, 177–78
Coconut Mayonnaise, 43–44
coconut meat, 2, 3, 6, **6,** 7, 9, 10–11
Coconut Meringue Bars, 180
coconut milk, 2, 3, 6, **6,** 7, 12–13, 17,
　19–21
Coconut Milk and Water Mix, 22
coconut milk beverage, 13

Coconut Milk Biscuits, 157
Coconut Milk–Fruit Smoothie, 32–33
Coconut Milk Pancakes, 149–50
Coconut Oatmeal, 155–56
Coconut-Oatmeal Cookies, 182
coconut oil, 1, 2, 3–6, **6**, 7, 10, 14–15,
     36–38
Coconut Oil, Toasted, 69
Coconut Oil Juice Mix, 39
Coconut Oil Miracle, The (Fife), 4, 5
Coconut Oil Pastry, 193–95
Coconut-Orange Banana Bread,
     161–62
Coconut-Orange Chicken, 103
Coconut-Orange Pancakes, 150
Coconut Pastry Shell, 195
Coconut-Peach Crisp, 209
Coconut-Pecan Bars, 183–84
Coconut-Pecan Frosting, 167
Coconut-Pecan Pie, 207–8
Coconut Pie, Frozen, 198–99
Coconut Pie, Super-Delicious, 198
Coconut-Pineapple Cake, 170–71
Coconut-Pineapple Ice Cream, 226–27
Coconut Pudding Squares, 217–18
Coconut-Raspberry Muffins, 147
Coconut Rice, 156
Coconut Rice, Indian-Style, 156–57
Coconut Rice Salad, 57
Coconut Sauce, 61
Coconut-Seafood Stew, 131–32
Coconut Sesame Balls, 189
Coconut Sherbet, 228
Coconut Shrimp, African, 113
Coconut Shrimp and Noodles, Thai, 127
Coconut Streusel Cake, 170–71
Coconut Sugar Cookies, 185–86
Coconut Tortilla Corn Chips, 144
Coconutty Muffins, 146
Coconutty Pancakes, 151
Coconut-Vanilla Ice Cream, Premium,
     223–24, 225, 226
Coconut-Vanilla Ice Cream, Quick,
     223, 224–25
Coconut-Vanilla Pudding, 215
coconut water, 2–3, 6, 7, 11–12, 21–22
Coconut Whipped Cream, 196–97
Coconut Whole-Wheat Pancakes, 149
cookies, 177–92
*Cooking with Coconut Flour: A Delicious
     Low-Carb, Gluten-Free Alternative
     to Wheat* (Fife), 10

corn
     Coconut–Corn Bread Muffins,
          148–49
     Coconut Tortilla Corn Chips, 144
     Corn and Potato Chowder, 86
     Corn Bread Dumplings, 93
     Corn Bread Muffins, 148–49
     Corn Chowder, 85–86
     Creamed Corn, 138–39
     Hush Puppies, 159
Crab Cheese Sauce, 63
Crab Chowder, 84–85
Crab Cups, 142–43
cracked coconuts, 7–8
Creamed Corn, 138–39
Creamed Peas, 139
Creamed Spinach, Spicy, 140
Creamed Vegetables and Fish Sauce,
     139–40
Cream Fillings for Cakes, 173–74
Cream of Artichoke Soup, 77–78
Cream of Asparagus Soup, 75
Cream of Broccoli Soup, 75–76
Cream of Cauliflower Soup, 76
Cream of Cauliflower Soup, Curried, 77
cream of coconut, 12
Cream of Mushroom Soup, 79
Cream of Potato Soup, 78–79
Cream of Spinach Soup, 78
Cream Pies, 199–200
Cream Puffs, 211–13
Creamy Cheese and Broccoli Soup,
     90–91
Creamy Cheese Sauce, 63
Creamy Chicken and Biscuits, 109
creamy coconut beverages, 22–28
     See also beverages
Creamy Coconut Dressing, 46
Creamy Fudge Ice Cream, 233
Creamy Mashed Potatoes, 136–37
Creamy Melon Salad, 50
Creamy Peach Smoothie, 36
Creamy Scalloped Potatoes, 135
Creamy Shrimp Linguine, 99
Creamy Tomato Soup, 80–81
Creamy Tomato-Vegetable Soup, 81
Creamy Tuna and Biscuits, 109–10
Creamy Zucchini Soup, 80
Crepes, 153
Crisps/Crispies (cookies), 189–90
Crisps (pies), 209
Croutons, 100

curry, 1, 117, 128
  Apple and Sweet Potato Curry,
    125–26
  Chicken in Curry Sauce, 119–20
  Chicken in Red Curry Sauce, 126
  Creamy Curry Dressing, 46
  Curried Cream of Cauliflower
    Soup, 77
  Curried Peas, 139
  Curry Gravy, 66
  Lamb and Squash Curry, 128–29
  Peach Curry, 53
  Pineapple Curry, 53
  Pork and Squash Curry, 128–29
  Potato and Spinach Curry, 130
  Red Thai Curry, 127–28
  Tossed Curry Salad, 52
custard
  Baked Custard, 219
  Black-Bottom–Custard Pie,
    203–4
  Coconut Custard Pie, 204
  Coconut Custard Sauce, 62
  Maple Custard, 219

dandruff, 2
Deluxe Clam Chowder, 83
desserts, 2
  See also cakes; cookies; ice cream;
    pies; puddings
digestible carbohydrates, 11
digestive problems, 2, 3, 36
dips. See flavored oils; gravies; salad
    dressings; sauces
Double Cheese Biscuits, 158
Double-Coconut Ice Cream, 226
Double Crust, 194, 195
dried coconut (shredded, grated,
    flaked), **6,** 9, 11, 17
dry sugars, 15
Dumplings, 74
Dumplings, Coconut, 133–34
Dumplings, Corn Bread, 93

Éclairs, 213
Eggnog, 26–27
egg yolk as emulsifier, 37–38
electrolytes in coconut water, 3, 12
emulsifier for adding coconut oil,
    37–38
energy, 4, 5, 36
"expeller pressed" coconut oil, 14, 15

fatigue, 2
fat in coconut, 3, 5, 12, 13
favorite recipes, 18
fiber in coconut (dietary fiber), 2,
    10–11
Fife, Bruce
  Coconut Ketogenic Diet, The, 5
  Coconut Oil Miracle, The, 4, 5
  *Cooking with Coconut Flour: A
    Delicious Low-Carb, Gluten-Free
    Alternative to Wheat,* 10
fish
  Catfish in Coconut Sauce, 106–7
  Coconut-Seafood Stew, 131–32
  Fish Chowder, 83
  Fried Sole with Coconut, 106
  Salmon in Coconut Cream Sauce, 105
  See also tuna
fish sauce, 63, 64, 85, 86, 99, 116
flaked (dried) coconut, **6,** 9, 11, 17
flavored oils, 68–71
  See also gravies; salad dressings;
    sauces
flavors for ice cream, 226–33
flour in recipes, 17
French Fries, 144
French Toast, 153–54
Fresh Fruit Coconut Oatmeal, 155
Fresh Fruit Ice Cream, 229
Fried Ice Cream, 232
Fried Mashed Potatoes, 136, 137
Fried Vegetables, 143–44
Fried Wonton Skins, 96
Fritters, Onion, 143–44
frostings
  Chocolate Frosting, 213
  Coconut Frosting, 166
  Coconut-Pecan Frosting, 167
  Orange Butter Frosting, 181
Frozen Chocolate Bananas, 233
Frozen Chocolate-Coconut Pie,
    198–99
Frozen Coconut Pie, 198–99
fruit
  Chocolate Fruit Smoothie, 34–35
  Fresh Fruit Coconut Oatmeal, 155
  Fresh Fruit–Flavored Milks, 22–25
  Fresh Fruit Ice Cream, 229
  Fruit and Coconut Cobbler, 210–11
  Fruit–Coconut Milk Smoothie,
    32–33
  Fruit Coconut Rice, 156

Fruit Cups, 142–43
Fruit-Flavored Ice Cream, 228
Fruit Sauce, 60–61
Fruit Sherbet, 227–28
Fruity Coconut Pancakes, 150
Fruity Tapioca Pudding, 220–21
Rice Pudding with Fresh Fruit, 218
Summer Fruit Salad, 51
sweetener in recipes, 16
Tropical Fruit Smoothie, 33
See also specific fruit
Fudge Ice Cream, Creamy, 233
full-sugar recipe versions, 15, 16

Garlic Cheese Sauce, 63
Garlic Mashed Potatoes, 136
Garlic Oil, 69
German Chocolate Cake, 166–67
Gingered Sweet Potatoes in Coconut
    Sauce, 129–30
Ginger Oil, 71
Ginger-Peach Shortcake, 174–75
Glaze, Lemon, 173
Glaze, Lime, 160
gluten sensitivity, 10
grains and breads, 17, 145–63
Granola, 154–55
Granola Bars, 190–91
grated (dried) coconut, **6**, 9, 11, 17
gravies, 64–67
    See also flavored oils; salad dressings;
    sauces
Green Beans and Potatoes in Coconut
    Sauce, 121–22
Green Star juicer, 20

Half and Half Pudding, 215, 217
Ham, Spinach, and Potato Casserole, 110
Ham and Potato Casserole, 110
Ham and Potato Soup, 88–89
Hawaiian Banana Bread, 161
Haystacks, 188
health food, coconut as, 1, 2–5, 36,
    37, 38
heart disease, 3, 4
Hearty Chicken Stew, 74
heated oils, 68–70
hemorrhoids, 2
hepatitis C, 4
Herbed Potato Salad, 54–55
Herb Oil, 71
herpes, 4

Homemade Coconut Milk and Cream,
    19–21
honey in recipes, 15, 17
Hot Chocolate, 25
Hush Puppies, 159

ice cream, 34–35, 223–33
ice cream makers, 223, 226
India, 3
Indian-Style Chicken/Lamb/Pork/
    Shrimp Stew, 118–19
Indian-Style Coconut Rice, 156–57
infections, 3, 4, 36
influenza, 2, 4
infused oils, 68, 70–71
Italian Dressing, 45
Italian Herb Oil, 71
IV solutions of coconut water, 2, 12

Japanese Vegetable Salad with Sesame
    Seed Dressing, 55–56
Jicama-Mango/Peach Salad, 54
Juice Blend, V-8, 41
Juice Mix, Coconut Oil, 39
Jumbo Fried Coconut Shrimp, 112

Kiwi Milk, 24
Korma, 123–24

Lamb and Squash Curry, 128–29
Lamb Stew, Indian-Style, 118–19
Lasagna, 100
lemon
    Lemon Chiffon Pie, 200–201
    Lemon Cream Filling for Cream
        Puffs, 212, 213
    Lemon Glaze, 173
    Lemon Mashed Potatoes, 136
    Lemon Meringue Pie, 205
    Lemon Oil, 70
Lentil (Red) Soup, 90
"light" coconut milk, 13
Lime-Coconut Pie, 206
Lime Glaze, 160
Linguine, Chicken or Creamy
    Shrimp, 99
liquid sweeteners, 15, 17
low-carbohydrate diets, 2, 10–11

Macaroni and Cheese, 142
Macaroons, 2, 177–78
main dishes, 1, 95–114

mangos
Jicama-Mango Salad, 54
Mango Dressing, 47
Mango Milk, 23
Mango Smoothie, 38
Powerhouse Mango Milk, 40–41
Zesty Mango-Banana Salad, 52
maple
Maple Custard, 219
Maple-Nut Ice Cream, 230
Maple Pudding, 215, 216
Maple Whipped Cream, 196–97
Marshmallow-Chocolate Swirl Ice
Cream, 231
Mashed Butternut Squash, 138
Mashed Potatoes, Creamy, 136–37
Mashed Sweet Potato, 138
Mayonnaise, Coconut, 43–44
MCTs (medium-chain triglycerides),
3, 4, 5
measles, 4
medium-chain triglycerides (MCTs),
3, 4, 5
Melon Salad, Creamy, 50
melting point of coconut oil, 14, 37
Meringue, 196
Meringue Bars, 180
Meringue Pies, 205–6
metabolism, 5, 36
Mexican Mashed Potatoes, 136
Mint, Chocolate, 26
moldy coconuts, 7, 8
mononucleosis, 4
muffins
Blueberry-Coconut Muffins, 147
Cherry-Coconut Muffins, 147
Cinnamon-Nut Muffins, 147–48
Coconut-Bran Muffins, 145–46
Coconut–Corn Bread Muffins,
148–49
Coconutty Muffins, 146
Corn Bread Muffins, 148–49
Raspberry-Coconut Muffins, 147
Mushroom à La King, 108, 109
Mushroom and Onion Cheese Sauce,
63, 64
Mushroom Soup, Cream of, 79

Nachos, Cheese, 144
nature's elixir. See coconut
New England Clam Chowder, 82
nondigestible carbohydrates, 11

noodles. See pasta
nuts
Cinnamon-Nut Muffins, 147–48
Coconutty Muffins, 146
Coconutty Pancakes, 151
Maple-Nut Ice Cream, 230
Nutty Chocolate Chip Cookies, 179
Pumpkin-Nut Bread, 162–63
See also almonds; peanut butter;
pecans

oat bran, 11
oats
Chocolate–Coconut-Oatmeal
Cookies, 182–83
Coconut Oatmeal, 155–56
Coconut-Oatmeal Cookies, 182
Fresh Fruit Coconut Oatmeal, 155
Onion Fritters, 143–44
Onion and Mushroom Cheese Sauce,
63, 64
Onion Oil, 69
opening a coconut, 8
oranges
Ambrosia, 48
Orange-Banana Salad, 50
Orange Butter Frosting, 181
Orange-Coconut Banana Bread,
161–62
Orange-Coconut Chicken, 103
Orange-Coconut Pancakes, 150
Orange Cream, 26
Orange Cream Delight, 227
Orange Dressing, 57
Orange Meringue Pie, 205–6
Orange Oil, 70
Piña Colada Fruit Drink, 24
Oyster Stew, 86–87

Pacific Islands, 3
pancakes
Baked Blueberry Pancake, 152
Baked Peach Pancake, 152
Coconut-Banana Pancakes, 151–52
Coconut Milk Pancakes, 149–50
Coconutty Pancakes, 151
Fruity Coconut Pancakes, 150
Orange-Coconut Pancakes, 150
Whole-Wheat Coconut Pancakes, 149
pasta
Almond Chicken with Noodles, 104
Asian-style cuisine and, 116

Beef Macaroni and Cheese, 142
Beef Stroganoff, 101–2
Chicken Linguine, 99
Creamy Shrimp Linguine, 99
Lasagna, 100
Macaroni and Cheese, 142
Shrimp and Pasta, 104–5
Thai Coconut Shrimp and
    Noodles, 127
Tuna Noodle Casserole, 102
Pastry, Pastry Shells, 193–95
peaches
    Baked Peach Pancake, 152
    Coconut-Peach Crisp, 209
    Creamy Peach Smoothie, 36
    Ginger-Peach Shortcake, 174–75
    Jicama-Peach Salad, 54
    Peach Curry, 53
    Peach Filling for Cobbler, 210
    Peach Salad, 51
    Peach-Yogurt Smoothie, 39–40
    Zesty Peach Smoothie, 33
peanut butter
    Burmese Peanut Chicken, 134
    Chocolate Peanut Butter Smoothie,
        34–35
    Peanut Butter–Apple Slaw, 53
    Peanut Butter Crispies, 189, 190
    Peanut Butter Pork, 130–31
    Peanut Chicken, 125
    substitution, 189
Peas, Creamed/Curried, 139
Pea and Potato Korma, 123–24
pecans
    Coconut-Pecan Frosting, 167
    Coconut-Pecan Pie, 207–8
    Pecan-Coconut Bars, 183–84
    Pecan Macaroons, 177
peppermint
    Peppermint Cream, 28
    Peppermint Cream Pie, 199, 200
    Peppermint Ice Cream, 230
    Peppermint Whipped Cream,
        196–97
pies, 193–213
Piña Colada Fruit Drink, 24
Piña Colada Smoothie, 35
pineapples
    Ambrosia, 48
    Coconut-Pineapple Ice Cream,
        226–27
    Piña Colada Fruit Drink, 24

Piña Colada Smoothie, 35
Pineapple-Banana Milk, 24
Pineapple-Coconut Cake, 170–71
Pineapple Curry, 53
Pineapple Macaroons, 177, 178
Pineapple Milk, 24
Pineapple Shrimp in Coconut Milk,
    124–25
Pineapple Smoothie, 39
pneumonia, 4
Polynesia, 4
Pork, Peanut Butter, 130–31
Pork and Squash Curry, 128–29
Pork Stew, Indian-Style, 118–19
potatoes
    Bacon and Cheese Potatoes, 136, 137
    Cheese and Potato Soup, 91
    Cheesy Mashed Potatoes, 136
    Corn and Potato Chowder, 86
    Cream of Potato Soup, 78–79
    Creamy Mashed Potatoes, 136–37
    Creamy Scalloped Potatoes, 135
    French Fries, 144
    Fried Mashed Potatoes, 136, 137
    Garlic Mashed Potatoes, 136
    Ham and Potato Casserole, 110
    Ham and Potato Soup, 88–89
    Herbed Potato Salad, 54–55
    Lemon Mashed Potatoes, 136
    Mexican Mashed Potatoes, 136
    Potato and Sausage Soup, 88
    Potato and Spinach Curry, 130
    Potatoes and Green Beans in
        Coconut Sauce, 121–22
    Potato and Pea Korma, 123–24
    Potato Salad, 54–55
    Potato Soup, 87
    Spinach, Ham, and Potato
        Casserole, 110
    Super Baked Potato, 137
    Twice-Baked Potato, 137–38
Potpies, 97–99
Powerhouse Mango Milk, 40–41
Premium Coconut-Vanilla Ice Cream,
    223–24, 225, 226
protein in coconut, 10
psoriasis, 2
Pudding, Yorkshire, 158–59
puddings, 215–21
Pumpkin-Nut Bread, 162–63
Pumpkin Pie, 207
Punch, Creamy Fruit, 25

Quick Chocolate Ice Cream, 231
Quick Coconut-Vanilla Ice Cream,
    223, 224–25
Quick Tartar Sauce, 60

Raisin-Cinnamon Rice Pudding,
    218, 219
raisins as natural sweetener, 31–32
Raspberry-Banana Salad, 49–50
Raspberry-Coconut Muffins, 147
recipe notes, 15–18
recommended amount of coconut oil,
    5–6, **6,** 36–37
Red Curry Sauce, 126
Red Lentil Soup, 90
Red Pepper Oil, 71
Red Thai Curry, 127–28
reduced-sugar recipe versions, 15–16
refined coconut oil, 14, 15
rice, 17, 218
    Almond Rice Pudding, 218
    Asian-style cuisine and, 116
    Brown Rice Pudding, 218
    Cardamom Rice, 141
    Chicken and Rice Stew, 89
    Chicken Rice Casserole, 107–8
    Cinnamon-Apple Rice Pudding,
        218, 219
    Cinnamon-Raisin Rice Pudding,
        218, 219
    Coconut Rice, 156
    Coconut Rice Salad, 57
    Fruit Coconut Rice, 156
    Indian-Style Coconut Rice,
        155, 156
    Rice Pudding with Fresh Fruit, 218
    Tuna Rice Casserole, 107–8
    Vanilla Rice Pudding, 218
ringworm, 4
Rocky Road Crisps, 189, 190
Rocky Road Ice Cream, 230–31

salad dressings, 1, 43–48
    See also flavored oils; gravies; sauces
salads, 1, 48–57
Salmon in Coconut Cream Sauce, 105
saturated fat, 3
Sauce, Coconut Cream, 105
Sauce, Red Curry, 126
sauces, 59–64
    See also flavored oils; gravies; salad
    dressings

sausage
    Potato and Sausage Soup, 88
    Sausage à La King, 108, 109
    Sausage Gravy, 66–67
    Spicy Sausage Gravy, 66–67
Scalloped Potatoes, Creamy, 135
Scones, 154
Seafood-Coconut Stew, 131–32
serving sizes, 17
sesame
    Coconut Sesame Balls, 189
    Sesame Chicken, 103–4
    Sesame Chicken Salad, 2, 55
    Sesame Seed Dressing, 47–48
    Sesame Seed Oil, 69
    Sesame Zucchini, 141
Shepherd's Pie, 111
Sherbet, 227–28
Shortcakes, 174–75
shredded (dried) coconut, **6,** 9, 11, 17
shrimp
    African Coconut Shrimp, 113
    Coconut Battered Shrimp, 111–12
    Creamy Shrimp Linguine, 99
    Indian-Style Shrimp Stew, 118–19
    Jumbo Fried Coconut Shrimp, 112
    Pineapple Shrimp in Coconut Milk,
        124–25
    Shrimp and Asparagus in Coconut
        Sauce, 113–14
    Shrimp and Cauliflower in Coconut
        Sauce, 122–23
    Shrimp and Pasta, 104–5
    Shrimp Cheese Sauce, 63, 64
    Shrimp Chowder, 84
    Shrimp Cocktail Drink, 30–31
    Shrimp Cups, 142–43
    Shrimp Macaroni and Cheese, 142
    Shrimp Oil, 70
    Thai Chicken and Shrimp Soup, 94
    Thai Coconut Shrimp and
        Noodles, 127
    Tomato-Shrimp Soup, 81–82
side dishes, 1, 135–44
Single Crust, 194, 195
sinus infections, 4
skin lesions, precancerous, 2
Slaw, Peanut Butter–Apple, 53
smoking point of coconut oil, 14
smoothies and blender drinks, 12, 22,
    31–41
    See also beverages

snacks, 1, 7
Snappy Tomato Juice Cocktail, 29–30
Sole (Fried) with Coconut, 106
Soup, Coconut-Chicken, 132
soups and chowders, 1, 73–94
South America, 3, 4
Southeast Asia, 3
South Pacific, 4
soybeans, 11
spices, sauces, and condiments,
    Asian-style cuisine, 115–16
Spicy Creamed Spinach, 140
Spicy Sausage Gravy, 66–67
spinach
    Cream of Spinach Soup, 78
    frozen vs. fresh, 78, 130, 132
    Potato and Spinach Curry, 130
    Spicy Creamed Spinach, 140
    Spinach, Ham, and Potato
        Casserole, 110
Sponge Cake, 172–73
Squash and Lamb Curry, 128–29
Squash and Pork Curry, 128–29
stevia, 15–16, 31
stews, 1
    Chicken and Rice Stew, 89
    Chicken and Sweet Potato Stew with
        Coconut Dumplings, 133–34
    Coconut-Seafood Stew, 131–32
    Hearty Chicken Stew, 74
    Indian-Style Chicken/Lamb/Pork/
        Shrimp Stew, 118–19
    Oyster Stew, 86–87
    See also soups and chowders
stir-fry dishes, 14
    Almond Chicken Stir-Fry, 96–97
    Beef Stir-Fry, 95–96
    Chicken Stir-Fry, 95–96
storage of coconut, 8, 9, 13, 14, 19
storage of flavored oils, 68
strawberries
    Strawberry-Banana Smoothie, 40
    Strawberry Chiffon Pie, 201–2
    Strawberry Ice Cream, 229
    Strawberry Milk, 22–23
    Strawberry Shortcake, 174–75
Streusel Coconut Cake, 170–71
Stroganoff, Beef, 101–2
sugar and sweeteners, 15–16, 17, 31–32,
    149, 189
Sugar Coconut Cookies, 185–86
Summer Fruit Salad, 51

Super Baked Potato, 137
Super-Delicious Coconut Pie, 198
super-healthy blender drinks, 36–41
    See also smoothies and blender drinks
Sweetened Coconut Milk, 21
sweeteners, 15–16, 17, 31–32,
    149, 189
sweet potatoes
    Apple and Sweet Potato Curry,
        125–26
    Chicken and Sweet Potato Stew
        with Coconut Dumplings,
        133–34
    Gingered Sweet Potatoes in Coconut
        Sauce, 129–30
    Mashed Sweet Potato, 138
    Sweet Potato Pie, 207

Tamale Soup, 92–93
Tapioca, 220–21
Tartar Sauce, 59–60
Tart Pastry Shells, 195
Tex-Mex Cheddar Cheese Sauce, 63
Tex-Mex Tomato Juice Cocktail, 30
Thai-style cuisine
    Red Thai Curry, 127–28
    Thai Chicken, 117–18
    Thai Chicken and Shrimp Soup, 94
    Thai Coconut Shrimp and
        Noodles, 127
Thick Cheddar Cheese Sauce, 63
Thousand Island Dressing, 44
thyroid function, 4
Toasted Coconut Oil, 69
Toffee–Chocolate Chip Ice Cream, 232
tomatoes
    Creamy Tomato Soup, 80–81
    Creamy Tomato-Vegetable Soup, 81
    Snappy Tomato Juice Cocktail,
        29–30
    Tex-Mex Tomato Juice Cocktail, 30
    Tomato Juice Cocktail, 29
    Tomato-Shrimp Soup, 81–82
toppings for pies, 196–97
Tortilla Coconut Corn Chips, 144
Tossed Curry Salad, 52
"Tree of Life," 4
    See also coconut, cooking with
Tropical Fruit Smoothie, 33
Tuna and Biscuits, Creamy, 109–10
Tuna Noodle Casserole, 102
Tuna Rice Casserole, 107–8

Turkey Calypso Salad, 56–57
Twice-Baked Potato, 137–38

U.S. Department of Agriculture, 11

V-8 Juice Blend, 41
vanilla
Basic Vanilla Cream Filling, 173–74
Coconut-Vanilla Pudding, 215
Premium Coconut-Vanilla Ice Cream,
223–24, 225, 226
Quick Coconut-Vanilla Ice Cream,
223, 224–25
Vanilla Cream, 28
Vanilla Cream Filling, Cream
Puffs, 212
Vanilla Cream Pie, 199
Vanilla Rice Pudding, 218
vegetable drinks, 28–31
Shrimp Cocktail Drink, 30–31
Snappy Tomato Juice Cocktail,
29–30
Tex-Mex Tomato Juice Cocktail, 30
Tomato Juice Cocktail, 29
See also beverages
vegetable oils vs. coconut oil, 14
vegetables
Chicken and Vegetables in Cream
Sauce, 120–21
Creamed Vegetables and Fish Sauce,
139–40
Creamy Tomato-Vegetable Soup, 81
Fried Vegetables, 143–44

Japanese Vegetable Salad with
Sesame Seed Dressing, 55–56
Vegetable-Beef Potpie, 98–99
Vegetables with Cheese Sauce, 141
See also specific vegetables
Vegetarian Gravy, 64–65
Vietnam, 12
Vinaigrette, 45
virgin coconut oil, 14, 15

Waldorf Salad, 48
wheat, 10, 11
Whipped Cream, 196–97
White Cream Gravy, 65
white spots in coconuts, 7–8
whole grains, 17
See also breads and grains
Whole-Wheat Coconut Pancakes, 149
Wonton Skins, Fried, 96
wontons substitution, 55
World War II, 12

Yogurt-Cherry Smoothie, 34
yogurt in smoothies and blender
drinks, 32
Yogurt-Peach Smoothie, 39–40
Yogurt Smoothie, 33–34
Yorkshire Pudding, 158–59

Zesty Mango-Banana Salad, 52
Zesty Peach Smoothie, 33
Zucchini, Sesame, 141
Zucchini Soup, Creamy, 80

ALSO BY BRUCE FIFE

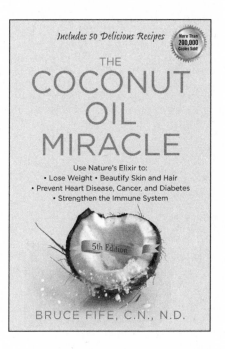

Get the completely revised and updated guide for maximizing the health and beauty benefits of coconut oil.